W0230360

Synthesis Lectures on Mechanical Engineering

This series publishes short books in mechanical engineering (ME), the engineering branch that combines engineering, physics and mathematics principles with materials science to design, analyze, manufacture, and maintain mechanical systems. It involves the production and usage of heat and mechanical power for the design, production and operation of machines and tools. This series publishes within all areas of ME and follows the ASME technical division categories.

Suchismita Satapathy ·
Tushar Kanta Mahapatra · Noe Alba-Baena ·
Meghana Mishra

Noise Pollution and Ergonomic Intervention by Acoustic Material

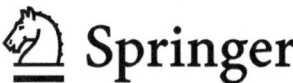 Springer

Suchismita Satapathy ⓘ
School of Mechanical Engineering
Kalinga Institute of Industrial Technology
Bhubaneswar, Odisha, India

Noe Alba-Baena
Universidad Autónoma de Ciudad Juárez
Ciudad Juárez, Mexico

Tushar Kanta Mahapatra ⓘ
School of Mechanical Engineering
Kalinga Institute of Industrial Technology
Bhubaneswar, Odisha, India

Meghana Mishra
School of Commerce and Economics
Kalinga Institute of Industrial Technology
Bhubaneswar, Odisha, India

ISSN 2573-3168   ISSN 2573-3176   (electronic)
Synthesis Lectures on Mechanical Engineering
ISBN 978-3-031-66307-9   ISBN 978-3-031-66308-6   (eBook)
https://doi.org/10.1007/978-3-031-66308-6

© The Editor(s) (if applicable) and The Author(s), under exclusive license to Springer
Nature Switzerland AG 2025

This work is subject to copyright. All rights are solely and exclusively licensed by the Publisher, whether the whole or part of the material is concerned, specifically the rights of translation, reprinting, reuse of illustrations, recitation, broadcasting, reproduction on microfilms or in any other physical way, and transmission or information storage and retrieval, electronic adaptation, computer software, or by similar or dissimilar methodology now known or hereafter developed.
The use of general descriptive names, registered names, trademarks, service marks, etc. in this publication does not imply, even in the absence of a specific statement, that such names are exempt from the relevant protective laws and regulations and therefore free for general use.
The publisher, the authors and the editors are safe to assume that the advice and information in this book are believed to be true and accurate at the date of publication. Neither the publisher nor the authors or the editors give a warranty, expressed or implied, with respect to the material contained herein or for any errors or omissions that may have been made. The publisher remains neutral with regard to jurisdictional claims in published maps and institutional affiliations.

This Springer imprint is published by the registered company Springer Nature Switzerland AG
The registered company address is: Gewerbestrasse 11, 6330 Cham, Switzerland

If disposing of this product, please recycle the paper.

Preface

This book includes six chapters, which focus on the physical, psychological, and mental stress of people suffering due to heavy noise in residential places and it was found that maximum noise was produced due to electronic appliances used by everyone in residential area. Even the noise from the neighbor's house is also distracting and people unable to focus on their work. Even sleeping disturbances, stress, anxiety, and behavioral changes were observed due to heavy noise. People also complained about fatigueless, headache, hair loss, breathlessness, and nerve issues due to high noise. In many cases, children, adults all suffering with partial or full hearing loss. Almost all over the world, noise is treated as pollution having an adverse effect on human health, like water and air pollution. Some noises are natural and some are human created. Natural noises occur due to volcanoes, due to spring, sea, rain, etc. But people make noises like shouting, quarrelling, high volume music, high frequency of machines, traffic, etc. Some are indoor noises and some are outdoor noises. Outdoor noises are traffic, train signals, crowd noise, machine noise, etc. Indoor noises are door or window clacking, pet barking, home appliances running, shouting, etc. People in residents want to take a rest after hard work the whole day, but the indoor noises of neighbors or their own place are very stressful for them. Unwanted sounds of home appliances are uncontrollable. It creates aggressiveness and helps to enhance to its peak during a bad mood, angry mood, and during alcohol drinking. The behavioral changes were marked due to unwanted noise.

To avoid unwanted noise, electronic appliances must be made noiseless, must be regularly maintained, must be used on plain surfaces, and sound-absorbing materials must be used, such that the unwanted noise can be absorbed, making the resident calm, quiet. Avoiding noise by using ear plugs has also negative impact on human health. People must use acoustic building materials in their floor, ceilings, and walls to filter the high noise of their home. Hence, use of acoustic noise-absorbing materials can avoid noise pollution and can keep people safer.

Hence, in Chap. 1, the detailed discussion about noise pollution and its effect on humans were discussed. Chapter 2 gives a clear concept of impact of noise and vibration on hearing impairments and measures were suggested to reduce indoor noise (electronic appliances' noise). Chapter 3 discusses the selection of acoustic materials and Chap. 4 provides a pictorial representation of all fabrication, testing procedures of acoustic materials. Chapter 5 discusses a few case studies, how to use acoustic materials to minimize noise effect and reduce noise pollution in residential areas. At the end, Chap. 6 concludes with sharing the importance of this research. It is an excellent guide for academicians and research scholars for postulating more innovative practices, framing policies, and designing devices to avoid noise pollution and for the extreme comfort of residential people.

Bhubaneswar, India   Suchismita Satapathy
Bhubaneswar, India   Tushar Kanta Mahapatra
Ciudad Juárez, Mexico   Noe Alba-Baena
Bhubaneswar, India   Meghana Mishra

About This Book

This book is based on the understanding and extensive use of information technology to explore noise-related risks in residential places due to noise. A framework is suggested through the systematic analysis of the barriers and their implementation, ergonomic analysis is performed to identify problems associated with hearing, and acoustic materials are fabricated and tested. Subsequently, a case study was conducted to reduce noise by placing acoustic material.

Contents

About the Authors

Suchismita Satapathy is an Associate Professor in the School of Mechanical Sciences, KIIT University, Bhubaneswar, India. She has published more than 130 articles in national and international journals, and conferences. She has published many books and e-books for academic and research purposes. Her areas of interest include production operation management, operational research, acoustics, sustainability, and supply chain management. She has filed three Indian patents, two of which have been published. She has more than 15 years of teaching and research experience. She has guided many Ph.D. (three completed and three ongoing), M.Tech. (20), and B.Tech. (49) students. She has published books such as Production Operation Management (Stadium Press) and MCDM methods for waste management with CRC Press; Innovation, Technology, and Knowledge Management with Springer; Soft Computing and Optimization Techniques for Sustainable Agriculture by DEGRUYTER; the PDCA cycle for industrial improvement; applied case studies by Springer; and many of her projects are ongoing.

Scopus Author ID: 55085975400

Tushar Kanta Mahapatra is a Lecturer at the KIIT Polytechnic in Bhubaneswar, Odisha, India. He is currently pursuing his Ph.D. in the School of Mechanical Engineering at KIIT, deemed to be a University in Bhubaneswar, India. He has published over 11 articles in national and international journals, conferences, and book chapters. His research interests include acoustic applications, production operation management, and ergonomics.

Scopus Author ID: 57220024588

Noe Alba-Baena is Professor (level "C") for the Department of Industrial and Manufacturing Engineering at the Universidad Autonoma de Ciudad Juarez (UACJ), Juarez, Mexico, January 2003–Present. Relevant accomplishments: During my 17-year professorship I guided me in graduating. More than 100 students (40 graduate students) focused on product design, automation, and process improvement, balancing this with industrial consulting, journal review, and international research laboratory experience.

Meghana Mishra is a Research Scholar in the School of Commerce in KIIT University, Bhubaneswar, India. She has published more than six articles in national and international journals, conferences, and book chapters. Her areas of interest include production operation management, economic study of the Agrisector, sustainability, business process reengineering, and ergonomics.

Abbreviations

AHP	Analytic Hierarchy Process
ANP	Atrial Natriuretic Peptide
ASTM	American Society for Testing and Materials
COPRAS	Complex Proportional Assessment
dB	Decibel
DEMATEL	Decision-Making Trial and Evaluation Laboratory
ELECTRE	Elimination and Choice Translating Reality
EVAMIX	Evaluation of Mixed Data
FA	Factor Analysis
GTMA	Grid Trade Master Agreement
HoQ	House of Quality
INRM	Influential Network Relationship Maps
IoT	Information of Technology
MCDM	Multi-Criteria Decision-Making
MOORA	Multi-Objective Optimization by Ratio Analysis
NRC	Noise Reduction Coefficient
OHS	Occupational Health and Safety
OSHA	Occupational Safety and Health Administration
PSI	Preference Selection Index
QFD	Quality Function Deployment
SAC	Sound Absorption Coefficient
SAW	Simple Additive Weighting
SWARA	Step-Wise Weight Assessment Ratio Analysis
TOPSIS	Technique for Order Performance by Similarity to Ideal Solution
TS	Thickness Swelling
UTM	Universal Testing Machine
WHO	World Health Organization
WPM	Weighted Product Model
WRTS	Waste Recycled Tire Steel

List of Figures

List of Tables

Noise Pollution by Electronic Appliances

1.1   Introduction

In recent years, the population has increased drastically and also modernization has changed Human life. In the home and office, people use many types of electronics appliances for their comfort and ease of completing a job. Electronic appliances used to complete our work within less time and in more sophisticated way than manual work. Hence, the demand for the use of electronic appliances is increasing day by day and, in the future, the requirement will be a more and more. These equipment/devices are the primary requirements for everyone. Even, it is very difficult to survive a day without the use of electronic gadgets. Appliances like a fridge, television, washing machine, air conditioners, heaters, grinders, food processor, micro oven, television and vacuum cleaner etc., are the basic gadgets found in almost all homes. Similarly, office laptops, air conditioners, heaters, personal computers, generators, printers, fax machines, telephones/mobiles etc. are very common. On one hand, with the use of electronic appliances, our work is done very easily without much labour. On the other hand, the noise generated from these gadgets during their use is very hazardous to human health. It not only affects our neighbors, animals, our ecosystem, but also effects on human health. Due to unwanted noise, headaches, sleeplessness, hearing.

Losses are very common symptoms. But sometimes this noise impacts on the physical and mental health of people and effects on behavioral changes and work efficiency/performance. Noise pollution has severe health effects like cardiac disorders, blood pressure etc. problems. It has a very negative impact on elderly people and also on small children. Noise is a way of expressing feelings, but the high noise is very disturbing and hazardous for health.

Noise can be controlled in many ways, by use of ear plugs, by reducing volume by use of a volume controller. By using sound absorbing materials in ceilings, walls and floors

© The Author(s), under exclusive license to Springer Nature Switzerland AG 2025

S. Satapathy et al., *Noise Pollution and Ergonomic Intervention by Acoustic Material*, Synthesis Lectures on Mechanical Engineering, https://doi.org/10.1007/978-3-031-66308-6_1

can also reduce noise pollution. Double glazed doors and windows can also reduce noise pollution. Keeping noisy appliances away from leaving place can control noise during work of electronic gadgets. Maintenance and repair of electronics appliances may help in reducing noise. Behavioral changes like playing less noise music, timely operating gadgets, low peach conversation etc. also help people from high noise.

Noise pollution has adverse effects on human health. As per the World Health Organization (WHO), a sound level more than 65 decibels (dB) is considered to be noise pollution. Noise is torturing over 75 decibels (dB) and hazardous above 120 dB. So, it is suggested to keep noise levels below 65 decibels during the day time, and during night time the ambient noise levels should be below 30 dB.

Noise can be categorized into different types depending on the frequency of the sound. Noise levels below 250 Hz are called low frequency noise, noise levels more than 2000 Hz is called high frequency noise. Electronic appliances produce different types of sound, sometimes humming, sometimes high noise and loud/high peak noise. Noise pollution from electronic appliances is very hazardous and difficult to bear for both residential and commercial environments. Radford et al. (2016) have discussed that noise pollution interrupts social connections and causes tension and anxiety in the observational group. Bala and Verma (2020) have discussed residential appliances and different sources of noise. Oishi and Schacht (2011) have discussed that noise pollution due to barking of dogs, playing of instruments by children are also disturbing. Jhanwar (2016) discussed about noise produced and also the level of noise.

Jariwala et al. (2017) have discussed the effect of noise pollution and its negative effect on human health and wellbeing. Berglund and Lindvall (2024) have explained that children are more sensitive to noise and more hearing damage than adults. Öztürk (1994) have discussed about the noise generating washing and cleaning machines. Sahdev and Sahu (2024) have studied about source of noise pollution in India and its effect on human health. Li et al. (2016) have found that houses hold appliances like blenders, pressure cookers etc. Hsu et al. (2012) have explained that the cause of hearing loss may be trauma, any diseases or may be exposure to heavy noise. Goines and Hagler (2007) have investigated that a sudden increase in noise can also generate negative responses in body like blood pressure, cardiovascular diseases. Singh and Davar (2004) have written that noise has both permanent and temporary effects on human body as well as mammals. Passchier-Vermeer and Passchier (2000) explained that alcohol, anger and aggressiveness will enhance more with noise. As High noise is very dangerous for small children, pregnancy women, and for all ages of people in society. So to study the impact of noise on human health is studied.

1.1.1 Research Methodology

To explore the effect of electronic appliances generated noise on human health, a standard set of questionnaires is designed and a survey is conducted in residential areas of Asian countries like India, Pakistan, China, Bangladesh, Nepal, Malaysia, Vietnam and Mexico etc. The inspection is conducted for 15–65 aged people of that residential area. Around 356 data was collected with personal contact, by phone, by mail and what's appall the 356 respondents were educated and the medium of communication was English for around 6–7 months (September 2023 to March 2024) time taken for data collection. Figure 1.1 shows the number of selected residential people of different countries. From Fig. 1.1 it was clear that maximum respondents were Indian and Mexico, as all collected data by authors with personal contact. The rest of the data was collected with the help of students, professors, and friends, relatives with personal contact, mail communication and by phone. As per Fig. 1.2a maximum no of respondent men were Indian and minimum males from Malaysia. Similarly, Fig. 1.2b shows that no of maximum female res-ponders were Indian and minimum Pakistan. All of them were using electronic appliances in their home. Figure 1.3 shows no users of electronic appliances among selected respondents and it was clear that a maximum of 356 respondents used mobile/phones in their homes and a number of respondents using a food processor was 103, which is the minimum the use of other appliances. Figure 1.4 shows respondents suffering with hearing problems due to the use of home appliances, and it was found that a maximum of 11 Indian respondents were suffering from hearing issues and a minimum of 2 Nepal respondents were suffering with hearing issue. It was found that a total of 47 people were suffering from hearing issues, not deaf from birth or had no hearing issues from child hood. Figure 1.5 shows gender wise hearing problem of respondents and it was seen that maximum female respondents were suffering with hearing problem. It was found that the maximum numbers of women 6 in Pakistan were suffering with hearing problems were non-working women and as per Fig. 1.6b maximum Indian and Bangladeshi non-working men were suffering with hearing issue. Hence, it was clear that hearing issues may be due to residential noise.

Fig. 1.1 Selected residential people of different countries

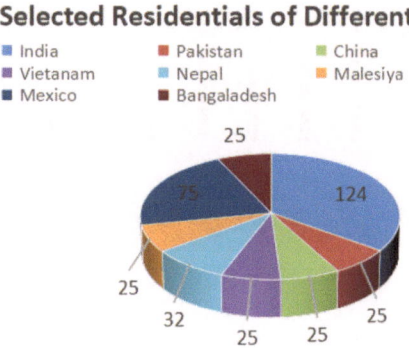

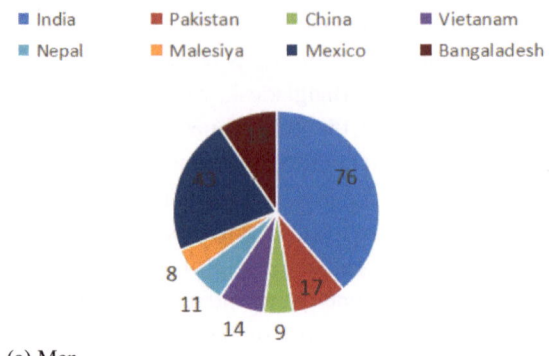

(a) Men

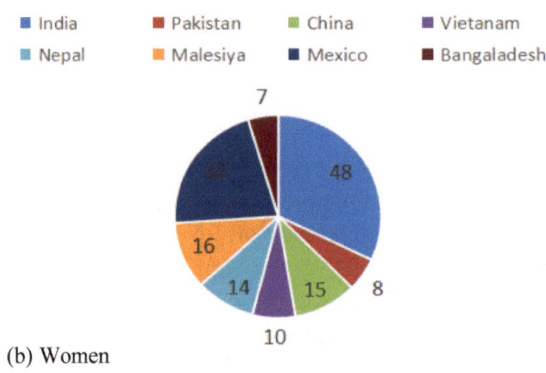

(b) Women

Fig. 1.2 **a** and **b** Selected residential women and men numbers

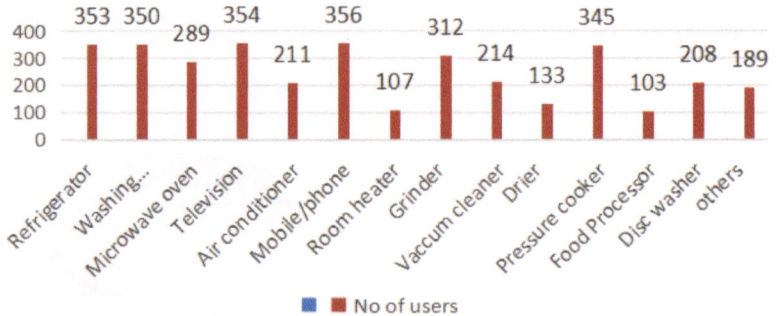

Fig. 1.3 Selected respondents using electronic appliances

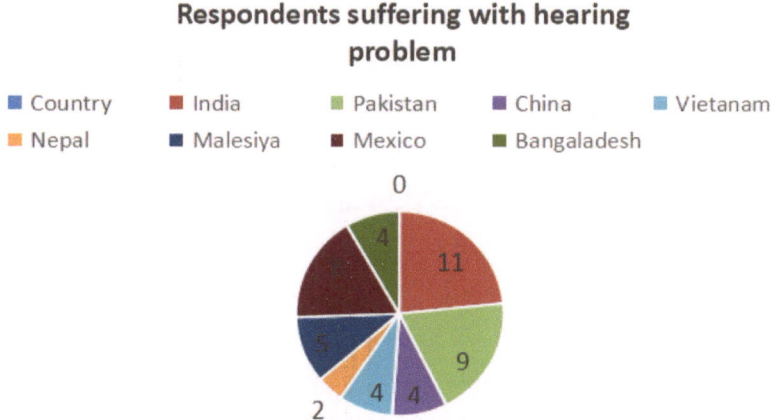

Fig. 1.4 Selected respondents suffering with hearing issues due to noise of electronic appliances

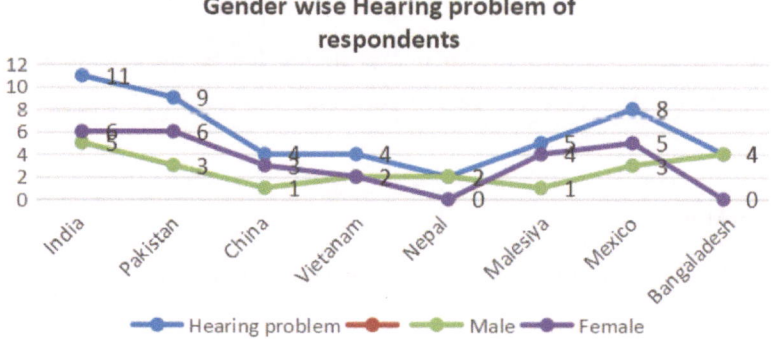

Fig. 1.5 Gender wise hearing problem

Table 1.1 shows age-wise hearing problems of men and women and it was seen that the maximum of 10 women of aged 55–65 and 6 men from 55 to 65 were suffering from hearing problems. After analyzing the selected respondents, the questionnaire (Table 1.2) was circulated and respondents were asked to answer in Likert scale (1–3) (1 = disagree, 2 = no opinion and 3 = agree). Then statistical analysis or factor analysis was conducted and health issues were prioritized to find the most important problem due to noise.

1.1.2 Results and Discussion

To find the effect of noise on human health, the collected data was analyzed by statistical software Minitab and factor analysis was conducted. Factor analysis was done to find

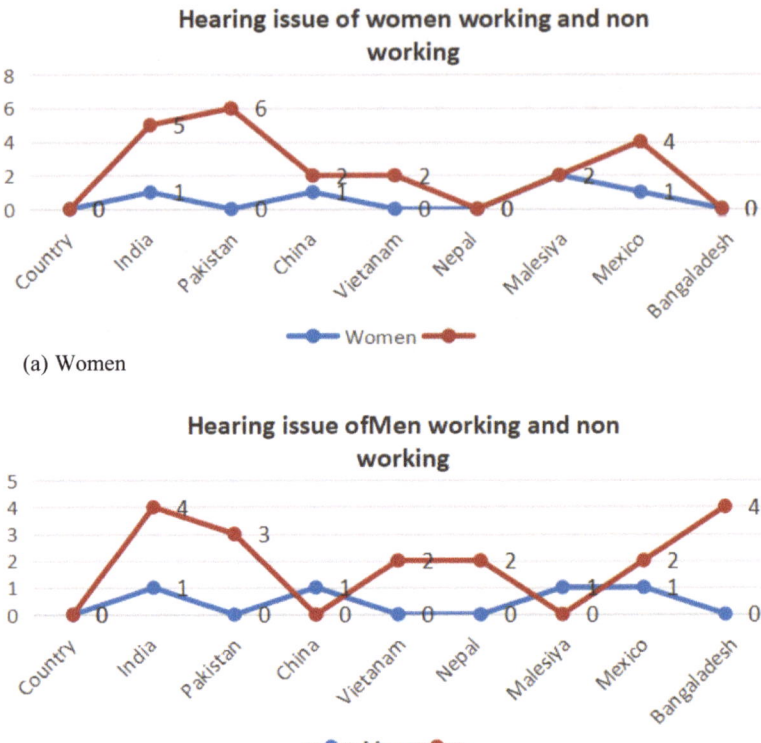

(a) Women

(b) Men

Fig. 1.6   a, b Hearing issue of women and men working and non-working

Table 1.1   Age wise hearing issues of men and women

Age	Hearing issue	
	Male	Female
0–15	1	1
15–25	2	1
25–35	4	3
25–45	4	5
45–55	4	6
55–65	6	10

similar and related variables in one cluster. The 15 variables whose chrobanch'alpha value more than 0.5 were selected under dimensions like Physical effect, psychological effect, behavioral change effect, Sleepless ness, work performance) etc. (Table 1.3). The variable having Chrobanch's alpha value less than 0.5 was discarded.

Table 1.2 Questionnaires for studying noise issues due to use of home appliances

Sl. no	Question	1	2	3	4	5
1	Sudden accidents	–	–	–	–	–
2	Mental stress	–	–	–	–	–
3	Sleep disturbance	–	–	–	–	–
4	Head ache	–	–	–	–	–
5	Hearing impairments	–	–	–	–	–
6	Speech interference	–	–	–	–	–
7	Lack of concentration	–	–	–	–	–
8	Annoyance	–				
9	Cardiovascular disturbances					
10	Restlessness					
11	Conflicts at home					
12	Blood pressure level changes					
13	Fatigue ness					
14	Breathing issues					
15	Lack of interest in work					
16	Nerve issues					

Table 1.3 Factor analysis

Dimensions	Items	Factor1	Factor2	Factor3	Factor4	Factor5
Physical effect	1,4,9 12,13, 16	0.501 0.512 0.529 0.589, 0.534 0.523				
Psychological effect	2,7		0.632 0.564			
Behavioral change effect	6,8 ,11			0.524 0.545 0.563		
Sleeplessness	3,4				0.529 0.574	
Work performance	5,15					0.612 0.643

Then a step-wise assessment ratio multi criteria decision making method was used to prioritize the effect of noise due to home appliances.

Tables 1.4, 1.5, 1.6, 1.7, 1.8 and 1.9 shows Swara analysis for factors and sub factors. From the Table 1.9, it was clear that the physical effect was maximum due to noise of electronic appliances. Table 1.10 shows Swara ranking of sub factors, and it was found that hearing impairments were mostly affected by noise due to home appliances, which is ranked first, then mental stress ranked second and sleep disturbances ranked third.

As noise of appliances is not constant, varying in nature with variation in frequency, so the noise produced is also difficult to measure, but the effects of noise pollution is very challenging. Hence, necessary actions must be taken by electronic appliance manufacturing companies to manufacture less noisy appliances and residents must do necessary

Table 1.4 Swara analysis for physical effect

Parameter	Comparative importance average value	Coefficient	Re-calculated weight	Final weight
Pj	Vj	Cj	Wj	Qj
P1		1	0.925925926	0.163743677
P4	0.08	1.08	1.009345794	0.178495911
P9	0.07	1.07	1.019047619	0.180211612
P12	0.05	1.05	0.882352941	0.156038092
P13	0.19	1.19	0.991666667	0.175369478
P16	0.2	1.2	0.826388889	0.146141231

Table 1.5 Swara analysis for psychological effect

Parameter	Comparative importance average value	Coefficient	Re-calculated weight	Final weight
Pj	Vj	Cj	Wj	Qj
P2		1	0.8	0.555555556
P7	0.25	1.25	0.64	0.444444444

Table 1.6 Swara analysis for behavioral change effect

Parameter	Comparative importance average value	Coefficient	Re-calculated weight	Final weight
Pj	Vj	Cj	Wj	Qj
P6		1	0.666666667	0.462857143
P8	0.5	1.5	0.444444444	0.308571429
P11	0.35	1.35	0.329218107	0.228571429

Table 1.7 Swara analysis for sleeplessness

Parameter	Comparative importance average value	Coefficient	Re-calculated weight	Final weight
Pj	Vj	Cj	Wj	Qj
P6		1	0.666666667	0.462857143
P8	0.5	1.5	0.444444444	0.308571429
P11	0.35	1.35	0.329218107	0.228571429
P3		1	0.909090909	0.523809524
P4	0.1	1.1	0.826446281	0.476190476

Table 1.8 Swara analysis for work performance

Parameter	Comparative importance average value	Coefficient	Re-calculated weight	Final weight
Pj	Vj	Cj	Wj	Qj
P5		1	0.571428571	0.636363636
P15	0.75	1.75	0.326530612	0.363636364

Table 1.9 Swara ranking for dimensions

Parameter	Comparative importance average value	Coefficient	Re-calculated weight	Final weight	Rank
Pj	Vj	Cj	Wj	Qj	
Physical		1	0.666666667	0.371949509	Ist
Psychological	0.5	1.5	0.444444444	0.247966339	2nd
Behavioral	0.3	1.3	0.341880342	0.190743338	3rd
Sleeplessness	0.6	1.6	0.213675214	0.119214586	4th
Work performance	0.7	1.7	0.125691302	0.070126227	5th

maintenance to reduce noise pollution. As per who, noise pollution has more effect on the environment, like water, air pollution. So, rules must be framed against noise in residential areas. More innovative research must be conducted to develop new building materials, new textiles and new machines to absorb noise. So that the health and mental issues due to noise pollution can be minimized.

Table 1.10 Final Swara ranking sub factors

Sub factors/variables	Weight	Rank	Name
P1	0.163743677	13th	Sudden accidents
P4	0.178495911	11th	Head ache
P9	0.180211612	10th	Cardiovascular disturbances
P12	0.156038092	14th	Blood pressure level changes
P13	0.175369478	12th	Fatigue ness
P16	0.146141231	15th	Nerve issues
P2	0.555555556	2nd	Mental stress
P7	0.444444444	6th	Lack of concentration
P6	0.462857143	5th	Speech interference
P8	0.308571429	8th	Annoyance
P11	0.228571429	9th	Conflicts at home
P3	0.523809524	3rd	Sleep disturbance
P4	0.476190476	4th	Headache
P5	0.636363636	Ist	Hearing impairments
P15	0.363636364	7th	Lack of interest in work

1.1.3   Conclusion

The total study imposes noise pollution and the physical and psychological stress due to it. The European Commission (1996) claims that noise has an impact on people's health, productivity, behavior, and well-being, some of the factors contributing to ambient noise exposure and its detrimental consequences on health are urbanization, economic expansion, and motorized transportation. Several factors, including industrial activity, music systems, construction, firecrackers, sound-producing instruments, loudspeakers, public address systems, vehicle horns, stone-crushing machines, defense equipment, televisions, refrigerators, generator sets AC, and other home appliances, are the reason for India's rising ambient noise levels in public spaces. So for the betterment and wellbeing of residential people, noise must be minimized or scaled up certain range by distinguishing day and night time. Social awareness, proper knowledge of noise and its detrimental effect on health may help to reduce noise to certain level.

References

Goines, L., & Hagler, L. (2007). Noise pollution: A modem plague. *The Southern Medical Journal, 100*(3), 287–294.

Hsu, T., Ryherd, E., Waye, K. P., & Ackerman, J. (2012). Noise pollution in hospitals: Impact on patients. *JCOM, 19*(7), 301–309

Jariwala, H. J., Syed, H. S., Pandya, M. J., & Gajera, Y. M. (2017). Noise pollution & human health: a review. *Indoor Built Environ, 1*(1), 1–4.

Jhanwar, D. (2016). Noise pollution: a review. *Journal of Environment Pollution and Human Health, 4*(3), 72–77.

Li, W. C., Tse, H. F., & Fok, L. (2016). Plastic waste in the marine environment: A review of sources, occurrence and effects. *Science of the Total Environment, 566*, 333–349.

Öztürk, C. (1994). Emitted noise levels of common home appliances used to clean and wash. *Building Acoustics, 1*(4), 299–312.

Passchier-Vermeer, W., & Passchier, W. F. (2000). Noise exposure and public health. *Environmental Health Perspectives, 108*(1), 123–131.

Radford, A. N., Lèbre, L., Lecaillon, G., Nedelec, S. L., & Simpson, S. D. (2016). Repeated exposure reduces the response to impulsive noise in European seabass. *Global Change Biology, 22*(10), 3349–3360.

Sahu, N. (2024). Noise pollution sources in India and their effect on human health. *Sustainability, Agri, Food and Environmental Research, 12*.

Singh, N., & Davar, S. C. (2004). Noise pollution-sources, effects and control. *Journal of Human Ecology, 16*(3), 181–187.

Prevalence of Discomfort with Hearing Due to Heavy Noise and Designing a Framework to Reduce the Noise Issues Due to Home Appliances

2

2.1 Introduction

Both indoor and outdoor noises were human life. The noise of traffic, machines, noise of music etc. were unwanted noises were faced by all aged people in their everyday life. These noises become the cause of hearing discomfort, some cases, partial or full hearing loss. Many people like to listen to music, if it is smooth in listening and does not disturb the ear or mind, it will be just like a cure to diseases. But the same music is disturbing and hazardous if the volume is high. When people are chatting with each other, it is not troublesome, but if they talk loudly, even on one side of the phone, it is disturbing. The noise of nature chipping of birds, fountains running, thunderstorms, heavy wind blowing, animals barking that are uncontrollable in nature, but man create noise, beeping sounds, humming sounds and running sound of machines can easily be controlled. Noise is essential and cannot be stopped, but control of noise according to social, ecological and human acceptable level will not be treated as pollution. This standard of noise will never harm others and will not be a cause of hearing loss also. Hence, it is reported that, exposure to sounds below 70 decibels does not cause hearing damage, regardless of time. Exposure to sound levels above 85 decibels (dB) for more than 8 h is generally considered harmful. Noise pollution is an unwanted or excessive noise that can harm human health, wildlife, and the environment. According to Buss (2007), (noise was 1st time acknowledged as a significant pollutant during the 1972 World Environment Congress in Stockholm. Subramani et al. (2012) have to say that the term "noise" refers to sound levels that are annoying and above reasonable limits. Regularly being in loud environments puts a great deal of stress on neurological and auditory systems. There are various causes of noise pollution, including both natural and human-made sources, which are exacerbated by urbanization and industrialization (Gupta et al., 2018). Non-industrial sources of noise include transportation/vehicular traffic as well as neighborhood noise caused by different

© The Author(s), under exclusive license to Springer Nature Switzerland AG 2025

S. Satapathy et al., *Noise Pollution and Ergonomic Intervention by Acoustic Material*,
Synthesis Lectures on Mechanical Engineering,
https://doi.org/10.1007/978-3-031-66308-6_2

types of pollution, which can be classified as natural, or manufactured (Singh & Davar, 2004).The use of power tools for gardening and home maintenance, such as lawnmowers and leaf blowers, can produce continuous loud noises that are commonly heard in residential neighborhoods, especially on weekends and during the summer (Huaang, 2006). Moreover, household appliances like vacuum cleaners, dishwashers, washing machines, and dryers also contribute to noise pollution when in use (Yolal et al., 2016).

Noise is a type of environmental pollution that affects people's quality of life; Noise pollution causes stress, which can lead to a variety of stress-related diseases including anxiety, depression, and a general decline in mental health (Freedman et al., 2001). Especially in urban places worldwide. In the current era of industrialization and technical growth, this has increased. According to the WHO 2018 report in the European Union, traffic noise affects at least 100 million people, and it claims that every year, 1.6 million people lose their lives due to this noise pollution. People in these loud urban regions appear to have grown because of the increased noise levels. The European Commission (1996) claims that noise has an impact on people's health, productivity, behavior, and well-being. Noise-induced hearing impairment can lead to aberrant loudness perception, distortion, and tinnitus. Tinnitus can be transient or develop permanent with prolonged exposure. Hearing loss can lead to loneliness, depression, speech discrimination, poor academic achievement, limited career options, and feelings of isolation (Passchier-Vermeer & Passchier, 2000). If noise levels are above this threshold, they pose a risk to the well-being and comfort of occupants. Those subjected to loud noises all day at work may sustain injuries such as hearing loss, nerve weakness, internal tissue soreness, cardiac difficulties, and persistently elevated blood pressure (Eggermont, 2017).

In Fig. 2.1, as per the Environment Protection Act (2002), noise level is standardized. The noise level for the residential areas must be 45 decibels during night time and not more than 55decibel during the daytime.

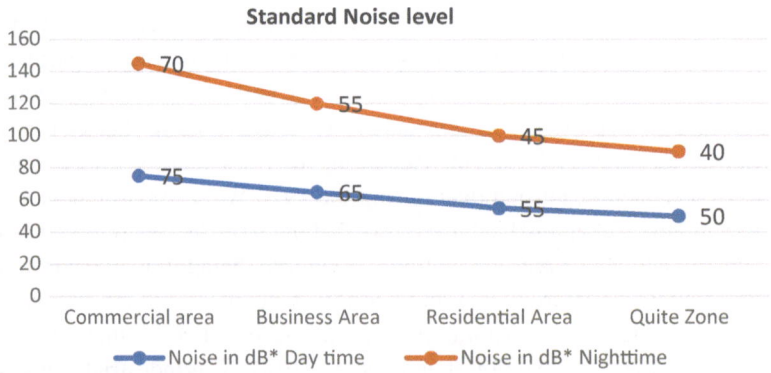

Fig. 2.1 Standard noise level

As daytime is the activity time and all household work is done, so the noise level in residential areas definitely increases. Hence, to avoid this high, noise awareness is required and also necessary steps must be taken during use of home appliances. New less noisy appliances must be used; repair and continuous maintenance of old equipment must be done. Use of building acoustics also absorbs sound at certain level and prevents noise from disturbing others.

Hence, in this chapter a framework is done to prevent noise pollution in residential areas and the discomfort of hearing is also measured.

2.1.1 Research Methodology

To study discomfort in the hearing level of residential people, an experiment was conducted among 124 Indians, Around 50 Indians were selected and those who had hearing issues were not included in this experiment. An Audiometry test was conducted with the help of medical/dispensary staff. All the selected residential were spent 8 to 10 h at home, maximum house wives, children and elderly people. All of them are either using electronic appliances or all home appliances were used in their place and also by their neighbors. Hearing discomfort was measured by audiometer device. Then regression analysis was conducted by considering independent variables such as sound and vibration of electronic appliances during working. A sound-measuring device (SL-4005) was used to measure the sound of different machines and units. In addition, a vibrometer was used to measure the vibrations of the different machines under average working conditions and. Table 2.1 show sound and vibration generated by home appliances. Figure 2.2 shows audiometer test of residents by medical staff.

2.1.2 Results and Discussion

Regression analysis was conducted by Minitab software. Sound (X_1) and vibrations (X_2) generated from home appliances were taken as independent variables and hearing impact was considered as dependent variable (Y). Below is equation is generated from regression analysis.

$$Y = 54.6 - 0.056X_1 - 1.37X_2 \qquad (2.1)$$

R square value is 7.7%, means it is a good fit. Fig. 2.2 shows graphs of residual fit.

Then a frame work is designed by quality function deployment to mitigate the adverse effect of noise due to appliances. Hence, a study is conducted to find the cause of noise in home appliances, called as customer requirement (What), and then the design requirement is suggested, called How to mitigate the noise problems in home appliances. Table 2.2

Table 2.1   Sound and vibration generated by electronic appliances

Sl no.	Home appliances	Sound in decibel (Average)	Average vibration	Hearing impact of residents
1	Refrigerator	43	4.84	42.32
2	Oven	50	2.92	45.32
3	Vacuum cleaner	76.5	3.2	51.42
4	Toaster	70	4.36	43.27
5	Dish washer	70.6	2.8	52.23
6	Washing machines	72.2	2.09	62.3
7	Electric kettle	80.8	1.56	31.42
8	Grinder	71.9	8.37	37.45
9	Cooker	44.4	6.3	36.36
10	Garbage disposal	66.6	5.78	42.36
11	Drier	71.9	6.24	48.45
12	Air conditioner	60	4.23	43.45
13	Room heater	43.2	5.46	34.64
14	Electric razor	79.8	2.2	39.10
15	Hair drier	70.9	2.4	38.20
16.	Lawn mower	90	3.8	45.20
17	Computer and printer	70	6.5	41.20
18	Extractor fan	58.5	3.9	59.40
19	Fan	45.5	3.6	56.50
20	Food processor	62.2	4.3	53.13

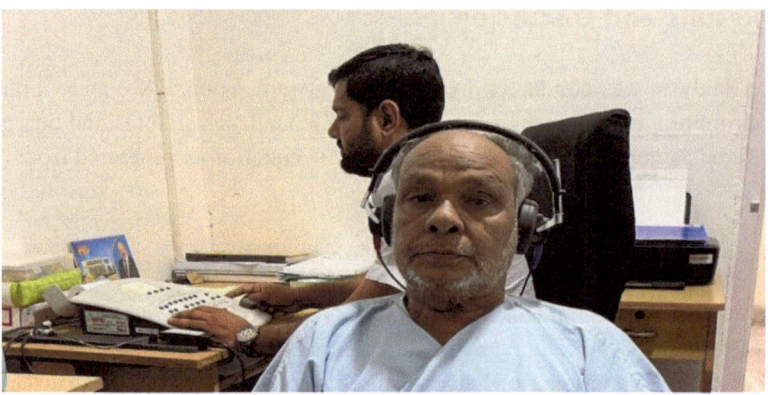

Fig. 2.2   Shows audiometer test of residents

shows the causes of noise generated in residential places, Table 2.3 shows how to mitigate the noise problem in residential areas. Table 2.4 and Fig. 2.4 shows House of quality.

From Fig. 2.4 and Table 2.4 it was found that use of noise absorbing materials around the appliances can reduce noise pollution is ranked first, Regular maintenance and checkup ranked 2nd and **Use of sound**-absorbing materials on walls and floors ranked 3rd.Hence, it was clear that materials with high sound-absorption coefficients are typically porous and called acoustic materials. By using these materials in the source of noise places like compressors, pumps, motors etc., noise can be reduced. Acoustic walls help reduce outside noise and keep residential people in safe condition.

Table 2.2 Cause of noise generated in residential places

Sl no.	Customer requirement
1.	During use of the washing machine, nose generated due to vibrations during spin cycles, mechanical components, and water flow
2.	During operating with refrigerator Compressor noise, fans, and defrost cycles
3.	Noise and vibration due to television and audio systems
4.	Kitchen appliances produce noise due to motor and mechanical parts
5.	In vacuum cleaner due to motor and air flow noise is produced
6.	In air conditioners and heaters, noise is produced due to compressors, air flow and fans
7.	In dishwasher, water flowing through pumps and motors produces noise
8.	Noise produced in some appliances during buzzing, operating for large time etc
9.	Old and broken appliances

Table 2.3 Design requirement

Sl no.	Design requirement
1	Use anti-vibration pads or mats under the appliance
2	Use sound-absorbing materials on walls and floors
3	Regular maintenance and check up
4	Clean the condenser coils and fans
5	Use noise absorbing materials around the appliances
6	In television audio system, control volume
7	Machine must be placed in proper level
8	Use soundproof boxes or enclosures while operating
9	Use of silicon mats to reduce noise

Table 2.4 House of quality for mitigating noise by home appliances

	requirement	1	2	3	4	5	6	7	8	9	Customer rating
1	1										7.538
2	4										13.846
3	2										8.954
4	3										12.553
5	2										6.276
6	1										7.538
7	5										6.276
8	1										4.384
Initial rating		55	60.55	59.21	56.71	63.76	53.58	49.87	50.06	53.21	
Revised Rating		35.55	43.81	47.63	39.1	54.2	29.54	38.65	43.53	41.1	
Normalized Rating		0.655904059	0.808302583	0.878782288	0.72140221 4	1	0.54501845	0.71309963 1	0.80313653 1	0.75830258 3	
Rank		8th	3rd	2nd	6th	1st	9th	7th	4th	5th	

2.1.3 Conclusion

Noise pollution is one of the invisible dangers of the other pollutants. It is present both on land and beneath water, even though it is invisible. Noise pollution is an unwanted or excessive noise that can harm human health, wildlife, and the environment. In particular, it is especially dangerous for kids, elderly people. Noise is the expression of life so it cannot be totally mitigated. It can be reduced but using sound absorbing materials in

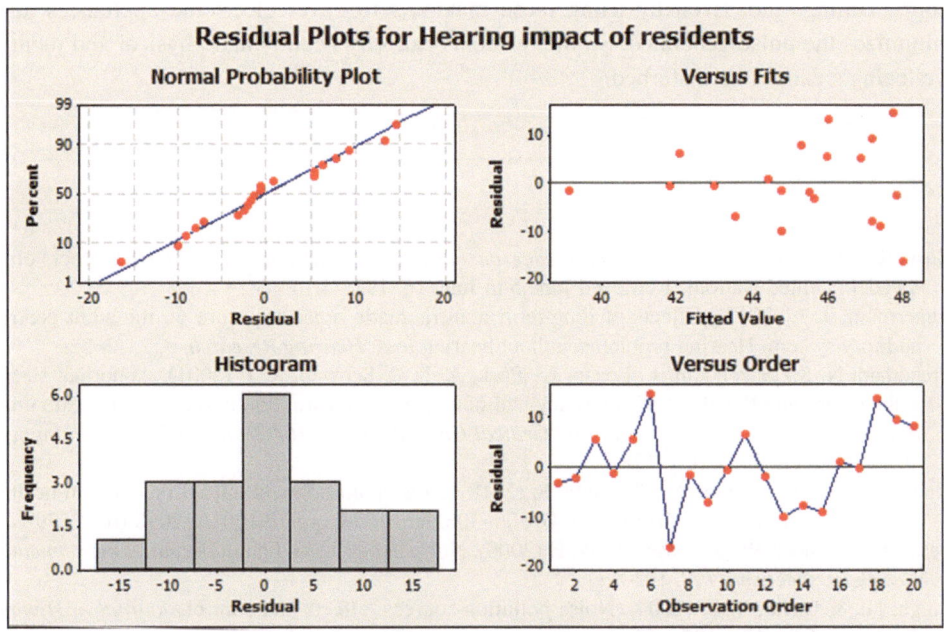

Fig. 2.3 Residual plots for hearing the impact of residential

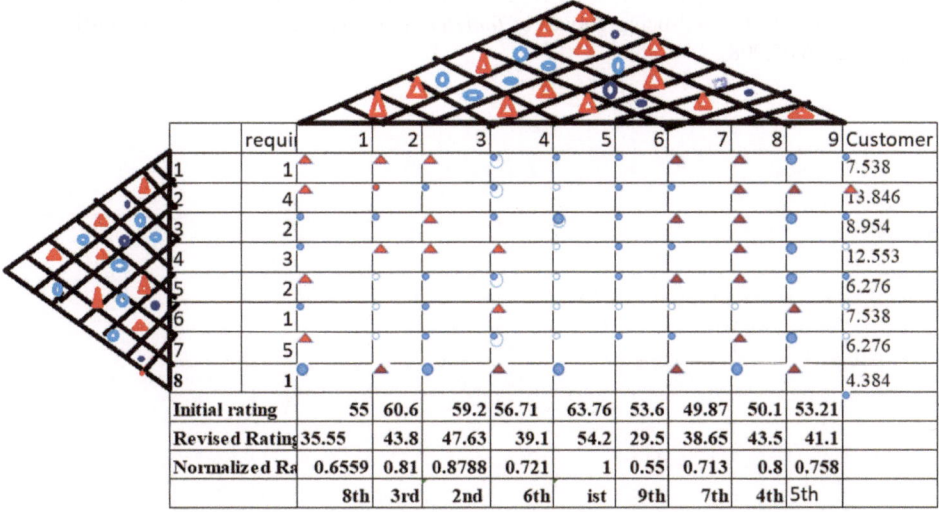

requi	1	2	3	4	5	6	7	8	9	Customer
1	1									7.538
2	4									13.846
3	2									8.954
4	3									12.553
5	2									6.276
6	1									7.538
7	5									6.276
8	1									4.384
Initial rating	55	60.6	59.2	56.71	63.76	53.6	49.87	50.1	53.21	
Revised Rating	35.55	43.8	47.63	39.1	54.2	29.5	38.65	43.5	41.1	
Normalized Ra	0.6559	0.81	0.8788	0.721	1	0.55	0.713	0.8	0.758	
	8th	3rd	2nd	6th	ist	9th	7th	4th	5th	

Fig. 2.4 HoQ for reducing noise due to electronic appliances

floors, ceilings etc. Even by using these materials to cover electronic appliances also minimizes the noise generated. So the residents can stay healthy and physical and mental wellbeing's cannot be disturbed.

References

Buss, R. (2007). *United Nations Conference on the Human Environment (UNCHE)*. Stockholm, Sweden: United Nations. Retrieved June 5 to June 16, 1972

Eggermont, J. J. (2017). Effects of long-term non-traumatic noise exposure on the adult central auditory system. Hearing problems without hearing loss. *Hearing Research, 352*, 12–22.

Freedman, N. S., Gazendam, J., Levan, L., Pack, A. I., & Schwab, R. J. (2001). Abnormal sleep/wake cycles and the effect of environmental noise on sleep disruption in the intensive care unit. *American Journal of Respiratory and Critical Care Medicine, 163*(2), 451–457. https://doi.org/10.1164/ajrccm.163.2.9912128

Gupta, A., Gupta, A., Jain, K., & Gupta, S. (2018). Noise pollution and impact on children health. *The Indian Journal of Pediatrics, 85*(4), 300–306. https://doi.org/10.1007/s12098-017-2579-7

Passchier-Vermeer, W., & Passchier, W. F. (2000). Noise exposure and public health. *Environmental Health Perspectives, 108*, 123–131.

Singh, N., & Davar, S. C. (2004). Noise pollution-sources, effects and control. *Journal of Human Ecology, 16*(3), 181–187.

Subramani, T., Kavitha, M., & Sivaraj, K. P. (2012). Modelling of traffic noise pollution. *International Journal of Engineering Research and Applications, 2*(3), 3175–3182.

Yolal, M., Gursoy, D., Uysal, M., Kim, H. L., & Karacaoğlu, S. (2016). Impacts of festivals and events on residents' well-being. *Annals of Tourism Research, 61*, 1–18. https://doi.org/10.1016/j.annals.2016.07.008

A Complete MCDM-Based Approach for Acoustic Material Selection Using the COPRAS Tool

3

3.1   Introduction

Many outdated materials have been changed in recent years by different advanced product in order to meet the requirement for weight reduction and improved associated qualities. The globe has around 80,000 materials, including metallic and nonmetallic materials for engineering use. Because of the various materials and intricate interactions between many selection qualities, evaluating and material selection for a particular technological use is sometimes a difficult and challenging subject to deal with. Material selection is a well-established conflicting problem in engineering design because it requires an understanding on various related properties like physical, electrical, mechanical, chemical, manufacturing, material cost, environmental effect, availability and other complicated relations between several picks. In Mechanical properties such as young's modulus, creep, fatigue, brittleness, ductility, hardenability, strength, yield stress, and toughness are observed, as well as physical properties such as density, colour, solubility, polarity, texture, and melting point, electrical properties, thermal properties such as specific heat, conductivity and diffusivity. Furthermore, studies and research are being conducted in order to develop new products with a variety of qualities as per the Chatterjee et al. (2009). Industry decision-makers must take into account different types of alternative features, including technical details, cost, aesthetics, serviceability, etc. Based on these considerations, a suitable alternative can be chosen as per the author Moradi (2023).

To comply with quality regulations and address quality-related issues in contemporary manufacturing processes, businesses must choose an inspection system, machine tools, the best design, process planning, materials, and so forth that are now offered. Making decisions is a difficult undertaking because a variety of factors might influence which alternative is best. According to Zavadskas et al. (2009) Material selection challenges and MCDM approaches have an unbreakable connection. The most difficult task

© The Author(s), under exclusive license to Springer Nature Switzerland AG 2025   21
S. Satapathy et al., *Noise Pollution and Ergonomic Intervention by Acoustic Material*,
Synthesis Lectures on Mechanical Engineering,
https://doi.org/10.1007/978-3-031-66308-6_3

in designing and developing new products is selecting appropriate materials. Over time, a material selection has drawn a lot of interest, due to the surge in new material development. Material selection is a complex decision-making process that includes choosing the best materials from a range of available choices based on a number of criteria. In general, material selection aims to decrease costs while satisfying customer requirements and performance goals. Furthermore, to make better decision-making, material selection must consider multiple attributes based on design requirements (Popovič et al., 2012). The enormous number of possibilities, combined with complicated relationships, affects the decision process for industrial designers, as these often demand stakeholders from other sectors to weigh in with their opinions in order to find the best suitable match for this application.

Consequently, any selection process aims to determine the best choice by considering all of its characteristics. Many methods, such as PSI (Preference selection index) "COPRAS, AHP" MOORA (multi-objective optimization by ratio analysis), EVAMIX (Evaluation of Mixed Data), SAW (Simple Additive Weighting), TOPSIS, DEMATEL, WPM (weighted product model), GTMA, ANP, ELECTRE (elimination and choice translating reality) and others, have recently been developed to address MCDM difficulties by Shyi-Ming (1997). To address the material selection problem, several MCDM strategies have been developed in the available literature.

However, a systematic and easy mathematical approach is required for efficient and effective evaluation and the finding of the best material with good sound absorption capabilities.

As we all know that Noise pollution is an undesired sound that is damped into the atmosphere without regard for the negative impacts it may have. Additionally, noise is defined as the incorrect sound at the incorrect location at the incorrect time. It is now the third largest cause of pollution and has a number of unavoidable negative impacts on the economy and human well-being. the author have Thakker et al. (2008) observed that noise also affects the work productivity and the health impact to the workers like hearing loss, sleep issue, cardiovascular and psycho-physiologic issues, and so on. Many countries are establishing strict noise pollution restrictions in response to the alarming growth in environmental noise pollution and accompanying health consequences. So selecting the best material for reducing this high noise by absorbing this sound is also a very difficult task for a human due to the increase in noise in our society.

The goal of this study is to look into the applicability and capabilities of a newly developed MCDM technique, the Complex Proportional Assessment (COPRAS) method, for selecting the best material for sound absorption. Until now, the COPRAS approach has had extremely limited application in material selection for this work.

3.1.1   Literature Review

In this subject, we will go across some relevant literature on MCDM methods to solve material selection problems, as well as how to select an MCDM technique. The literature review is divided into two sections: (i) The study on the effects of noise on people and (ii) Studies on the different MCDM methods and the application of the COPRAS method.

(i) **The study on the effects of noise on people**

Nowadays, noise pollution is not an unusual problem for the average person, particularly in the majority of industrial towns and large cities. Any sound that the recipient finds objectionable is considered noise pollution. The frequency of sound determines how it affects humans. It is well known that human ears can detect sounds in a very broad frequency range, ranging from 0 to 180 dB. Human activity produces noise in a variety of ways. Pantawane et al. (2017) suggest that noise is the result of an inappropriate sound occurring at an inappropriate time and place. Unwanted noise that is spread across Noise pollution is defined as the release of sound into the environment without regard for the potential harm it may create. According to the author Jariwala et al. (2017), noise pollution is a big issue in the city area all over the world. Except for that which originates in the workplace, ecological trouble consists of a large number of unwanted sounds in our networks. Workers on the manufacturing line are subjected to high levels of noise as a result of the hardware used on a regular basis. Srivastava (2014) states that the sounds that is louder than 65 decibels (dB) is called noise pollution as per the WHO report. Any noise level beyond 75 decibels (dB) is dangerous, and any noise level above 120 dB is uncomfortable. Therefore, daily noise levels should be maintained at or below 65 dB. When nighttime noise levels rise above 30 dB, it might also be difficult for a human for night's sleep.

According to Panhwar et al. (2018), noise has a negative impact on human wellbeing's and can affects the hearing issues such as nerve weakness and problems with hearing, as well as other issues such as less efficiency, irritation, Heart-related issues, hypertension, and many more. In addition, sound causes headaches, impatience, anxiety, and weariness, which, when combined with the other variables discussed above, may lead to more serious and long-term health concerns. Many researchers are involved in the study of selection difficulties. There is a wealth of literature available on the application of decision-making procedures for selecting from several choices and qualities. For the quantitative assessment of complex economic or social processes, multicriteria approaches have become more popular recently (Kpang & Dollah, 2021) shows that noise has a detrimental effect on health and can lead to a variety of problems, including anxiety, heart problems, high blood pressure, and auditory problems such nerve exhaustion and partial hearing loss. Researchers (Kahya, 2007) claims that noise poses a risk to the health and safety of workers in the industrial safety and health sector. According to Münzel et al. (2014), noise is a stress-mediator that impairs sleep, focus, and communication in addition to altering psycho-social behaviour and usually resulting in substandard performance in daily tasks. The most common symptoms of noise are also linked to elevated heart rate, severe hypertension, physiological disturbances, and peripheral vascular resistance, according to author Jariwala et al. (2017). According to Kamble et al. (2022) the development of a risk assessment approach for managing the efficient components appears to be urgently necessary for vital infrastructures, irrespective of the weighted relative value of the assessment criteria. Using a theoretical framework, the effect of the physical work environment on employee performance was examined. The five main factors that affect employee performance are temperature, sound, air quality, light and colour, and the actual physical area of the workplace. So it clearly shows from the above literature review that noise is an unwanted sound that may affect human beings as well as society.

(ii) **Studies on MCDM methods and the application of the COPRAS method**

As per Ishizaka and Siraj (2018) and Baydaş et al. (2022) the term "Multi-Criteria Decision Making" (MCDM) refers to a group of techniques whereby potential solutions are compared against a number of frequently at odds criteria, such as certain weighting schemes, in an effort to determine which option is best. MCDM techniques are widely utilized to condense various, occasionally contradictory performance aspects of businesses into a single performance outcome as per Diakoulaki et al. (1995). Jahan et al. (2010) suggested a linear assigning technique for ordering engineering materials for a specific engineering component based on numerous characteristics. Multiple criteria for financial performance analysis are measured, according to De Almeida-Filho et al. (2021), using Multi-Criteria Decision Making (MCDM) methodologies. Because of this, the MCDM paradigm effectively provides a final compromise answer as opposed to offering an acceptable solution that takes into account several factors. Evaluating a company's financial performance is a crucial task for decision-makers since it shows managers, investors, and shareholders the firm's advantages over rivals as well as its shortcomings as per Zopounidis and Doumpos (2002).

The suggested method for choosing materials was rather straightforward and was able to address issues with choosing materials that had to do with user interactions or qualitative qualities. A GTMA material selection method was developed by Rao (2008) for a particular engineering component. Many material selection factors were taken into consideration, together with their relative importance for the application in question, to create a digraph. Rao and Davim (2015) developed a suitable material selection strategy for a specific engineering design using TOPSIS and AHP methodologies. The decision-maker might assess and rank the materials using the recommended material selection index. Jahan et al. (2010) evaluated quantitative strategies developed to handle choosing materials difficulties for various engineering components. These methods' specifics, application modalities, benefits, and shortcomings were mainly discussed. On the other hand, Shanian and Savadogo (2009) utilized the ELECTRE (Elimination and Choice Expressing Reality) technique to make a highly accurate material selection for a specific application. They also developed a material selection decision matrix and conducted criterion sensitivity analysis. Jee and Kang (2000) used two decision-making theories to rank the candidate materials and choose the best material for a flywheel: (a) TOPSIS (method for ordering preference by similarity to ideal solution), which uses entropy to determine the weight of each material feature. Chan and Tong (2010) proposed a combined method for selecting materials using grey relational analysis. This approach, which included an end-of-life product plan and an ordered pair of materials, was designed to help decision-makers assess and rank different kinds of materials. The suggested material selection index was designed to help with this process.

The COPRAS technique has been widely used in literature. In essence, COPRAS (Complex Proportional Assessments) is an MCDM technique that determines the ideal-worst solution and a ratio with the ideal-worst solution to identify the best option from a set of feasible solutions in (1996) by Zavadskas and Kaklauskas. Various researchers use this technique to solve decision-making challenges. Madić et al. (2014) designed the COPRAS technique to address a manufacturer's selection challenge for a manufacturer of agriculture and construction equipment. The COPRAS-generated rankings of alternative suppliers have been compared to those provided by earlier researchers. When choosing a provider, cost, durability, delivery performance, distance, and supply variation were all considered. Popovic et al. (2012) used the COPRAS and COPRAS-G methods to solve an investment project selection problem based on financial attributes and the usage of erroneous data. Average Rate of Return, Profitable Index, Project Level Risk, Pay Back Period, and Net Current Value were used as project selection criteria. From among the list of competitors, the best project was chosen using the COPRAS and COPRAS-G (COPRAS-Grey) systems. For the social media platform selection problem in a fuzzy environment, Tavana et al. (2013) have suggested a hybrid model that integrates fuzzy set theory, ANP, and the COPRAS-G technique. Vujičić et al. (2016) used the COPRAS approach to select the best compact fluorescent bulb from a group of available lamps. The following factors were evaluated while selecting a light: brightness, total perceived power, as well as active power, cost of the product, and lamp life. For a specific manufacturing company, Mulliner et al. (2013) evaluated a number of residential places' affordability based on social, environmental, and economic factors. The fuzzy COPRAS algorithm has been employed by Çakir and Özdemir (2018) to select the best six sigma projects from a list of eleven possibilities. In their study, Bayrakci and Aksoy (2019) compare the results of companies that manage assets for individual pensions, which are regarded as long-term investment tools, to the Additive Ratio Assessment and COPRAS approaches. COPRAS and ARAS were used by Chatterjee and Chakraborty (2013) to tackle a gear material selection problem. The following factors were used to choose the gear materials: ultimate tensile strength, bending failure, and core hardness.

Zavadskas et al. (2001) created the COPRAS technique to examine the building phases of life and choose the optimal solution. A home credit access model was created by Zavadskas et al. (2004) using the COPRAS methodology. Kaklauskas et al. (2006) examined the work of the window replacement contractors for the main building of Vilnius Gediminas Technical University. With the COPRAS technique, Kaklauskas et al. (2007) choose the optimum building choice. Zavadskas et al. (2004, 2007) recommended analyzing road design alternatives using the COPRAS approach. Kaklauskas et al. (2007) used the COPRAS approach to assess the market value of real estate. Chatterjee and Chakraborty (2013) used the COPRAS approach to determine which Flexible Manufacturing System (FMS) would be best for a certain organization. Following a review by Jahan et al. (2010), COPRAS and EVAMIX were examined for the material selection. Comparing COPRAS to AHP and EVAMAIX, they stated that it is a simpler method and requires less time to calculate. Banaitiene et al. (2008) calculated a structure's life cycle using the COPRAS approach. Using the COPRAS methodology, Viteikien and Zavadskas (2023) assessed the environmental sustainability of residential areas in Vilnius City. A hybrid approach was put forth by Liou et al. (2016) to address the confusing information provided by decision-makers and the dependent interactions between various criteria.

A straightforward and exacting mathematical procedure is still needed to enable the decision-maker to choose the optimal material for a given technical application, although earlier academics have conducted a substantial study on material selection utilizing a range of MCDM methodologies. In this work, an effort is made to evaluate the usefulness and potential of contemporary MCDM techniques, particularly the complex proportional assessment (COPRAS) technic for choosing the optimum material for a specific engineering work. This MCDM approach has only a few applications in the engineering field as of yet.

3.1.2 Methodology

3.1.2.1 COPRAS Method

Vilnius Gediminas Technical University researchers created the complex proportional assessment preference ranking system (COPRAS) in 1996. The impact of maximizing and minimizing criteria on the evaluation outcome is addressed independently in this method. It implies that the importance and usefulness level (priority) of the options depend directly and proportionally by the authors Chatterjee and Chakraborty (2014). To make the best decision, both ideal and impractical options are taken into account. The COPRAS approach, used in this instance to locate appropriate acoustic material, uses a sequential process for ranking and assessing the alternatives according to their relevance and usefulness level. Both the criteria i.e. (beneficial and non-beneficial), can be examined individually during this process, can be taken into consideration by the COPRAS technique. The COPRAS method's capacity to determine the utility degree of alternatives which reveals How much one choice differs from other alternatives used as a benchmark is what sets it apart from other approaches.

The case study will be considered in order to put the proposed COPRAS technique to the test. Efforts to rank diverse materials for usage as the best sound-absorbing materials for construction materials, as well as increased public demand, exacerbate the problem. The COPRAS technique starts the problem-solving process by building a decision matrix and determining how much weight to assign each criterion. The following phases are another approach that can be utilized to address concerns with Multicriteria decision-making using the COPRAS method.

1. Get started by reviewing the literature.
2. Collection of Data
3. Find out both the Beneficiary criterion and Non-beneficiary criterion.
4. Uses the COPRAS Method to compute the data.
5. Setting up the system
6. Select the best value from the data set.
7. Complete the approach by ranking the materials.

The COPRAS method employs the following phases. It is first believed that the issue has 'm' options and 'n' requirements (Chatterjee & Chakraborty, 2013):

Step 1:

The linear normalization approach to develop the normalized decision matrix:

$$r_{ij} = \frac{X_{ij}}{\sum_{i=1}^{m} X_{ij}} (i = 1, 2 \ldots m; j = 1, 2 \ldots n) \tag{3.1}$$

Zavadskas et al. (2009) prior to comparison, the criteria's values should be normalized if they are measured in different ways. In the Eq. (3.1), X_{ij} and r_{ij} stand for the ith alternative's performance in reference to the jth criterion and its normalized value, respectively.

Step 2:

The following factors are weighted in the normalized decision-making matrix (D):

$$D = \left[d_{ij}\right]_{m \times n} = r_{ij} \times w_j \tag{3.2}$$

The total of each criterion's dimensionless weighted normalized values determines its weight in all cases.

$$\sum_{i=1}^{m} d_{ij} = w_j$$

where w_j represents the important weight for the jth criterion. For evaluate the importance of criteria, several weighing methods can be used to obtain weights.

Step 3:

Each beneficial and non-beneficial criterion's weighted normalized score is added together.

$$S_{+i} = \sum_{j=1}^{n} d_{+ij}$$

$$S_{-i} = \sum_{j=1}^{n} d_{-ij} \qquad (3.3)$$

The both the criteria i.e. (beneficial and non-beneficial criteria) weighted normalized values are d_{+ij} and d_{-ij}, respectively. The additions of both the criteria are always equal to the addition of S_{+i} and S_{-i}, respectively, by using below following formulae.

$$\sum_{i=1}^{m} S_{+i} = \sum_{i=1}^{m} \sum_{j=1}^{n} d_{+ij}$$

$$\sum_{i=1}^{m} S_{-i} = \sum_{i=1}^{m} \sum_{j=1}^{n} d_{-ij}$$

Step 4:

The following formula is used to determine each option's relative weights or priority (Qi):

$$Qi = S_{+i} + \frac{S - \min \sum_{i=1}^{m} S - i}{S - i \sum_{i=1}^{m} (S - \min / S - i)} \qquad (3.4)$$

$$= S_{+i} + \frac{\sum_{i=1}^{m} S - i}{S - i \sum_{i=1}^{m} (1/S - i)}$$

S_{-i}'s smallest vale is $S_{-\min}$. The relative importance value of different alternative indicates how satisfied that alternative is. The importance of the alternative increases with Qi value, the optimal choice is the option with the highest relative significance value (Qmax) among the different alternatives.

Step 5:

The quantifiable utility (Ui) value of every option is assessed. By contrasting the priorities of each alternative with the most effective one, it is possible to determine an option's level of utility, which is then represented as follows:

$$U_i = \left[\frac{Qi}{Q\max} \right] 100\% \tag{3.5}$$

where Q_{max} = the highest value of relative importance. The options' utility values are in a range between 0 and 100%.

This technique makes it possible to evaluate the utility and relevance of the many examined alternatives, as well as the weights and performance values of the chosen alternatives, with respect to all of the criteria in a scenario where multiple criteria need to be taken into consideration.

3.1.3 Case Study

According to the assessment of the literature, numerous research projects have already been completed by earlier researchers to address material selection issues utilizing various MCDM-based techniques, but few work has yet been done to compare the corresponding outcomes of various multi-criteria approaches while addressing the issues with material choices (i.e. for selection of sound absorbing material). A contextual investigation will be considered as a means of testing the COPRAS technique shown. Making materials that can lessen the excess noise produced by various sources, including small businesses, the automotive industry, etc. This case study primarily determines the various mechanical and thermal properties of various sound-absorbing materials (biodegradable and Non-biodegradable) and develops a structure to determine their ranking order for those properties. These materials are easily available in our surroundings at reasonable cost. Due to their favorable qualities, a total of 12 materials (Table 3.1) including jute, wood, sugarcane, cotton, rice husk, rice etc. have been taken into account. Tensile strength, tensile modulus, and Young's modulus are beneficial characteristics among these six criteria, while density, diameter, and heat conductivity are non-beneficial characteristics where lowest values are preferred.

3.1.4 Result and Discussion

In order to compare all of these criteria when using the COPRAS technique to address this sound-absorbing material selection problem, the data from the option matrix, is initially

Table 3.1 For different properties of materials

Sl. no	Types of materials	Tensile strength (Mpa)	Tensile modulus (Gpa)	Young's modulus	Diameter(μm)	Density (g/cm³)	Thermal conductivity
M1	Bamboo	441	35.9	10	240	0.91	0.55
M2	Wood	78	2.35	9500	10	1.5	0.12
M3	Rice paddy	69.72	2.42	204.5	3.47	1.152	0.082
M4	Luffa	19.5	28	1332	250	0.61	0.206
M5	Coconut fiber	3.1	2.3	1465	69	1.4	0.168
M6	Jute	800	13	30	25	1.5	0.42
M7	Cotton	597	5.5	3.7	14	1.52	0.243
M8	Rice husk	135	0.3	2.6	60.54	0.67	0.08
M9	Sugarcane	400	6.42	18.81	200	1.25	0.119
M10	Sea grass	453	3.1	4.1	5	1.5	0.42
M11	Banana trunk waste	161.8	8.5	27	100	0.8	0.249
M12	Waste tire crumb	25	0.3	0.01	1	1.2	0.5
		Beneficial			Non-beneficial		

transformed into dimensionless values using a linear normalization technique, as illustrated in Table 3.2, Eq. (3.1) is then used to determine the related weighted normalized matrix (Table 3.3).

As shown in Table 3.4, the weighted normalized values for the S_{+i} (beneficial) and S_{-i} (non-beneficial) attributes are now added together using Eq. (3.3).

The relative importance value (Q_i) for individual alternative sound-absorbing material is then calculated using formula (3.4), as shown in below Table 3.5. That table provides the quantitative utility (U_i) value for every alternative, which is derived from formula (3.5) and used to generate a comprehensive ranking of the alternatives.

Suitable materials are sorted from highest to lowest U_i values for the sound absorption material selection problem, giving a thorough ranking of the materials as Material $_{12}$ (waste tire crumb) > Material $_{11}$ (banana) > Material $_{10}$ (sea grass) > Material $_9$ (sugar cane) > Material $_8$ (rice husk) > Material $_7$ (cotton) > Material $_6$ (jute) > Material $_5$ (Coconut fiber) > Material $_4$ (Luffa) > Material $_3$ (rice paddy) > Material $_2$ (wood) > Material $_1$ (bamboo). Material $_{12}$ (waste tire crumb) is the best option, whereas material M_1 (bamboo) is the poorest. In this case, the ranking of options is determined by the decision-makers assessment of the relative relevance of each alternative in comparison to

Table 3.2 Normalized decision matrixes

Step 2: normalized decision matrix

1	0.1113	0.2716	0.0007	0.2364	0.0009	0.0005
2	0.0197	0.0178	0.6784	0.0099	0.0015	0.0001
3	0.0202	0.0183	0.0454	0.0034	0.0011	0.0001
4	0.0058	0.2118	0.3098	0.2463	0.0006	0.0002
5	0.0009	0.0174	0.4937	0.0680	0.0014	0.0002
6	0.2386	0.0983	0.0200	0.0246	0.0015	0.0004
7	0.2339	0.0416	0.0025	0.0138	0.0015	0.0002
8	0.0690	0.0023	0.0018	0.0596	0.0007	0.0001
9	0.2198	0.0486	0.0128	0.1970	0.0012	0.0001
10	0.3190	0.0235	0.0028	0.0049	0.0015	0.0004
11	0.1673	0.0643	0.0187	0.0985	0.0008	0.0002
12	0.0310	0.0023	0.0000	0.0010	0.0012	0.0005

Table 3.3 Weighted normalized decision matrix

Types of material (M)	Step-3: weighted normalized decision matrix					
1	0.0278	0.0679	0.0002	0.0591	0.0002	0.0001
2	0.0049	0.0044	0.1696	0.0025	0.0004	0.0000
3	0.0051	0.0046	0.0114	0.0009	0.0003	0.0000
4	0.0014	0.0530	0.0775	0.0616	0.000 2	0.0001
5	0.0002	0.0043	0.1234	0.0170	0.0003	0.0000
6	0.0597	0.0246	0.0050	0.0062	0.0004	0.0001
7	0.0585	0.0104	0.0006	0.0034	0.0004	0.0001
8	0.0173	0.0006	0.0004	0.0149	0.0002	0.0000
9	0.0549	0.0121	0.0032	0.0493	0.0003	0.0000
10	0.0797	0.0059	0.0007	0.0012	0.0004	0.0001
11	0.0418	0.0161	0.0047	0.0246	0.0002	0.0001
12	0.0078	0.0006	0.0000	0.0002	0.0003	0.0001

the others. The decision-maker's decision will deviate from the recommended ranking if they alter the weights or relative relevance.

Table 3.4 The sums of weighted normalized values

Types of material (M)	S_{+i}	Value	S_{-i}	Value
1	S_{+1}	0.0959	S_{-1}	0.0595
2	S_{+2}	0.2748	S_{-2}	0.0623
3	S_{+3}	0.2958	S_{-3}	0.0635
4	S_{+4}	0.4277	S_{-4}	0.1253
5	S_{+5}	0.5557	S_{-5}	0.1426
6	S_{+6}	0.6449	S_{-6}	0.1493
7	S_{+7}	0.7144	S_{-7}	0.1532
8	S_{+8}	0.7327	S_{-8}	0.1683
9	S_{+9}	0.8030	S_{-9}	0.2179
10	S_{+10}	0.8893	S_{-10}	0.2196
11	S_{+11}	0.9519	S_{-11}	0.2444
12	S_{+12}	0.9602	S_{-12}	0.2451

Table 3.5 Q_i and U_i values for alternative materials

Types of material (M)	Q_i	U_i	Rank
1	0.512863	24.58145	12
2	0.730634	35.01917	11
3	0.818042	39.20859	10
4	0.746886	35.79813	9
5	0.858969	41.17025	8
6	0.955362	45.79034	7
7	1.040139	49.85365	6
8	1.055519	50.59082	5
9	1.07381	51.46753	4
10	1.166508	55.91052	3
11	1.210741	58.03058	2
12	1.221342	58.5387	1

3.1.5   Conclusion

The primary issue of the MCDM, choosing the optimal sound absorption material, was resolved using the COPRAS approach and the pertinent data CRITIC weighting technique. The data acquired from academic studies was used to calculate the weighting objective of the criteria. When using this technic, it is beneficial to examine and priorities choice possibilities. The amount of elective by comparing the variation under consideration, utility is established to the best one in a perfect environment. It might be stated that the proportion with an ideal option could be used when attempting to rank other possibilities and develop methods of working on an elective assignment. In this paper, we give a successful example of how multi-criteria decision making may be utilized to successfully select the optimum material for sound absorption techniques. Regarding calculations and rankings of the different choices waste tire crumb with the tensile strength 25 Mpa, tensile modulus 0.3 Gpa, Young's Modulus 0.1, diameter 1 μm, thermal conductivity 0.5, and density 1.2 b/cm^3 shows the best result among other considered alternatives. Among other alternatives Banana trunk waste shows the 2nd best and bamboo shows the shows the poorest.

The method makes sense when applied to both qualitative and quantitative data since it can effectively handle arbitrary numbers of options and attribute data. It should also be highlighted that the proposed strategy is considerably simpler and logical in comparison to others in this category. The suggested method is applicable to any sort of selection and decision-making challenge. Any parameters or alternatives that are simply eliminated must be recreated and evaluated due to how easily they can be changed.

References

Almeida-Filho, A. T. D., de Lima Silva, D. F., & Ferreira, L. (2021). Financial modelling with multiple criteria decision making: A systematic literature review. *Journal of the Operational Research Society, 72*(10), 2161–2179.

Banaitiene, N., Banaitis, A., Kaklauskas, A., & Zavadskas, E. K. (2008). Evaluating the life cycle of a building: A multivariant and multiple criteria approach. *Omega, 36*(3), 429–441.

Bayrakci, E., & Aksoy, E. (2019). Comparative performance assessment with entropy weighted ARAS and COPRAS methods of private pension companies. *Business and Economics Research Journal, 10*(2), 415–433.

Baydaş, M., Elma, O. E., & Pamučar, D. (2022). Exploring the specific capacity of different multi criteria decision making approaches under uncertainty using data from financial markets. *Expert Systems with Applications, 197*, 116755.

Çakir, E., & Özdemir, M. (2018). Alti sigma projelerinin bulanik copras yöntemiyle değerlendirilmesi: bir üretim işletmesi örneği. *Verimlilik Dergisi*, (1), 7–39.

Chan, K. S., & Tong, H. (2010). A note on the invertibility of nonlinear ARMA models. *Journal of Statistical Planning and Inference, 140*(12), 3709–3714.

Chatterjee, P., & Chakraborty, S. (2013). Gear material selection using complex proportional assessment and additive ratio assessment-based approaches: A comparative study. *International Journal of Materials Science and Engineering, 1*(2), 104–111.

Chatterjee, P., Athawale, V. M., & Chakraborty, S. (2009). Selection of materials using compromise ranking and outranking methods. *Materials & Design, 30*(10), 4043–4053.

Diakoulaki, D., Mavrotas, G., & Papayannakis, L. (1995). Determining objective weights in multiple criteria problems: The critic method. *Computers & Operations Research, 22*(7), 763–770.

Ishizaka, A., & Siraj, S. (2018). Are multi-criteria decision-making tools useful? An experimental comparative study of three methods. *European Journal of Operational Research, 264*(2), 462–471.

Jariwala, H. J., Syed, H. S., Pandya, M. J., & Gajera, Y. M. (2017). Noise pollution & human health: A review. *Noise and Air Pollutions: Challenges and Opportunities, Ahmedabad: LD College of Eng.*

Jahan, A., Ismail, M. Y., Mustapha, F., & Sapuan, S. M. (2010). Material selection based on ordinal data. *Materials & Design, 31*(7), 3180–3187.

Jee, D. H., & Kang, K. J. (2000). A method for optimal material selection aided with decision making theory. *Materials & Design, 21*(3), 199–206.

Kaklauskas, A., Zavadskas, E. K., & Trinkunas, V. (2007). A multiple criteria decision support on-line system for construction. *Engineering Applications of Artificial Intelligence, 20*(2), 163–175.

Kahya, E. (2007). The effects of job characteristics and working conditions on job performance. *International Journal of Industrial Ergonomics, 37*(6), 515–523.

Kamble, A. G., Kalos, P. S., Mahapatra, K., & Bhosale, V. A. (2022). Selection of raw material supplier for cold-rolled mild steel manufacturing industry. *International Journal for Simulation and Multidisciplinary Design Optimization, 13*, 16.

Kpang, M. B. T., & Dollah, O. C. (2021). Monitoring noise level in cities: A step towards urban environmental quality management in Nigeria. *World Journal of Advanced Research and Reviews, 10*(3), 348–357.

Liou, J. J., Tamošaitienė, J., Zavadskas, E. K., & Tzeng, G. H. (2016). New hybrid COPRAS-G MADM Model for improving and selecting suppliers in green supply chain management. *International Journal of Production Research, 54*(1), 114–134.

Madić, M., Marković, D., Petrović, G., & Radovanović, M. (2014, June). Application of COPRAS method for supplier selection. In *The Fifth International Conference Transport and Logistics-TIL 2014, Proceedings* (pp. 47–50).

Maniya, K. D., & Bhatt, M. G. (2013). A selection of optimal electrical energy equipment using integrated multi criteria decision making methodology. *International Journal of Energy Optimization and Engineering (IJEOE), 2*(1), 101–116.

Moradi, N. (2023). *Multi-criteria evaluation and ranking of circular economy water management alternatives for Porsuk Basin* (Master's thesis, Middle East Technical University).

Mulliner, E., Smallbone, K., & Maliene, V. (2013). An assessment of sustainable housing affordability using a multiple criteria decision making method. *Omega, 41*(2), 270–279.

Münzel, T., Gori, T., Babisch, W., & Basner, M. (2014). Cardiovascular effects of environmental noise exposure. *European Heart Journal, 35*(13), 829–836.

Pantawane, P. B., Dhanze, H., Verma, M. R., Singh, G., Kapdi, A., Chauhan, J., & Bhilegaonkar, K. N. (2017). Seasonal occurrence of Japanese encephalitis vectors in Bareilly district, Uttar Pradesh, India. *Journal of Vector Borne Diseases, 54*(3), 270–276.

Panhwar, M. A., Memon, D. A., Bhutto, A. A., & Jamali, Q. B. (2018). Impact of noise pollution on human health at industrial site area Hyderabad. *Indian Journal of Science and Technology, 11*, 1–6.

Popovič, A., Hackney, R., Coelho, P. S., & Jaklič, J. (2012). Towards business intelligence systems success: Effects of maturity and culture on analytical decision making. *Decision Support Systems, 54*(1), 729–739.

Popovic, G., Stanujkic, D., & Stojanovic, S. (2012). Investment project selection by applying COPRAS method and imprecise data. *Serbian Journal of Management, 7*(2), 257–269.

Rao, R. V., & Davim, J. P. (2008). A decision-making framework model for material selection using a combined multiple attribute decision-making method. *The International Journal of Advanced Manufacturing Technology, 35*, 751–760.

Rao, R. V. (2008). A decision making methodology for material selection using an improved compromise ranking method. *Materials & Design, 29*(10), 1949–1954.

Shanian, A., & Savadogo, O. (2009). A methodological concept for material selection of highly sensitive components based on multiple criteria decision analysis. *Expert Systems with Applications, 36*(2), 1362–1370.

Shyi-Ming, C. (1997). A new method for tool steel materials selection under fuzzy environment. *Fuzzy Sets and Systems, 92*(3), 265–274.

Srivastava, A. K. (2014). Noise: A nauseating nuisance for human life. *ZENITH International Journal of Multidisciplinary Research, 4*(2), 212–221.

Tavana, M., Momeni, E., Rezaeiniya, N., Mirhedayatian, S. M., & Rezaeiniya, H. (2013). A novel hybrid social media platform selection model using fuzzy ANP and COPRAS-G. *Expert Systems with Applications, 40*(14), 5694–5702.

Thakker, A., Jarvis, J., Buggy, M., & Sahed, A. (2008). A novel approach to materials selection strategy case study: Wave energy extraction impulse turbine blade. *Materials & Design, 29*(10), 1973–1980.

Vujičić, M., Blagojević, M., & Papić, M. (2016). Application of COPRAS MCDM method for choosing the best compact fluorescent lamp. In *International Scientific Conference, University of Kragujevac* (pp. 71–74).

Zavadskas, E. K., & Kaklauskas, A. (1996). Pastatų sistemotechninis įvertinimas.

Zavadskas, E. K., Kaklauskas, A., & Kvederytė, N. (2001). Multivariant design and multiple criteria analysis of a building life cycle. *Informatica, 12*(1), 169–188.

Zavadskas, E. K., Kaklauskas, A., & Gulbinas, A. (2004). Multiple criteria decision support web-based system for building refurbishment. *Journal of Civil Engineering and Management, 10*(1), 77–85.

Zavadskas, E. K., Kaklauskas, A., Peldschus, F., & Turskis, Z. (2007). Multi-attribute assessment of road design solution by using the COPRAS method. *The Baltic Journal of Road and Bridge Engineering, 2*(4), 195–203.

Zavadskas, E. K., Kaklauskas, A., & Vilutiene, T. (2009). Multicriteria evaluation of apartment blocks maintenance contractors: Lithuanian case study. *International Journal of Strategic Property Management, 13*(4), 319–338.

Zopounidis, C., & Doumpos, M. (2002). Multicriteria classification and sorting methods: A literature review. *European Journal of Operational Research, 138*(2), 229–246.

Thermal, Mechanical and Sound Absorbing Characterization of Waste Material (Recycle Waste Tire Crumb/Epoxy Resin/Hardener) Reinforced Hybrid Composite

4

4.1 Introduction

With the advancement of modern industrial and transportation systems, increase of pollutions like noise, soil, air, water and the increase of waste (Tire, Textile, Plastic) are affecting human health and the environment globally as per Mashaan and Karim (2014). Among these pollution it is well known that noise pollution, particularly in big cities, has been gradually impacting people all over the world. So to limit the effects of noise pollution has become a serious concern for human beings. The question of how to lessen noise-related damage has grown significantly. Generally speaking, noise can be managed in two ways. Abdulhameed et al. (2022) have explained that the first is to reduce or eliminate noise sources by designing buildings with reduced or no noise. Although this approach is useful, the technology available today typically does not allow it to control every source of noise. Utilizing materials for sound insulation and absorption is the second method, which allows the sound wave to be reduced or completely removed during transmission.

Similarly increases of urbanization the producer of waste are also increasing day by day. According to World Bank research, the world generates 2.01 billion tonnes of municipal solid garbage yearly; at least 33% of it is not managed in an environmentally responsible manner. The average daily amount of trash produced per person varies greatly around the world, ranging from 0.11 to 4.54 kg. High-income nations contribute more than 34%, or 683 million tonnes, of the rubbish produced globally, despite making up only 16% of the global population. So increase of waste is big concern for storage and dumps. If we see the below graph (Fig. 4.1) by 2050 It's predicted that waste will reach 3.40 billion tonns worldwide. However, the fastest growing regions are Sub-Saharan Africa, South Asia, the Middle East, and North Africa; by 2050, it is estimated that the total amount of rubbish created in these countries will more than triple, double, and quadruple,

© The Author(s), under exclusive license to Springer Nature Switzerland AG 2025
S. Satapathy et al., *Noise Pollution and Ergonomic Intervention by Acoustic Material*,
Synthesis Lectures on Mechanical Engineering,
https://doi.org/10.1007/978-3-031-66308-6_4

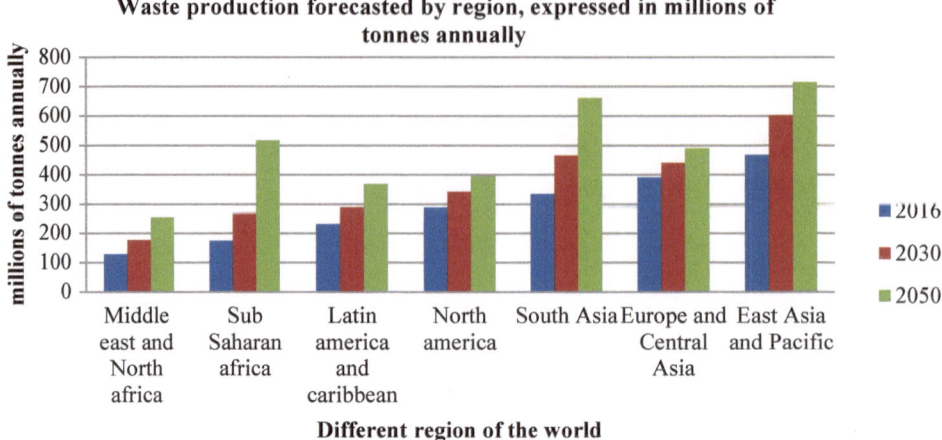

Fig. 4.1 Production of waste by different region from the world (Aoudia et al., 2017)

respectively. As the majority of waste in these places is dumped outdoors, prompt action is required to halt the waste's trajectory, which could have detrimental impacts on the environment, public health, and economic development.

As per Murgel (2007) There are different types of waste are producing from our society and these are electronic waste, waste tire, Textile waste, Medical waste etc. According to the World Bank database maximum waste produced from the food and green products but these are basically biodegradable, easily dump and not that much harmful to the human beings. But total 31% wastes are come from rubber, tire, leather and plastic, which are non-biodegradable in nature and harmful to the human beings (Fig. 4.2). These wastes are basically used for land filling, recycle and other related work. But that is not sufficient. So it's necessary to reuse and do them in other useful work so that we can produce a healthy and clean environment.

As the author Khaloo et al. (2008) have mentioned that among all the waste End-of-life-tires (Waste tires) is one of the major waste. To recycle and recover raw materials, the

Fig. 4.2 Percentage data on global waste in a year (2005–2009 report)

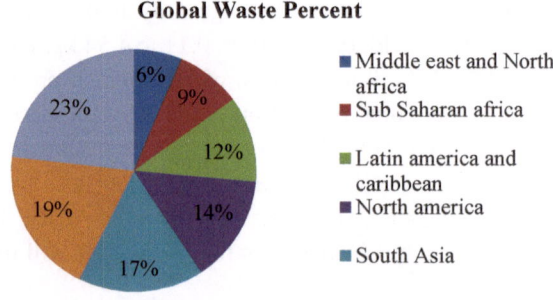

Fig. 4.3 Use of the waste tire in the different purpose U.S scarp tire disposition 2017

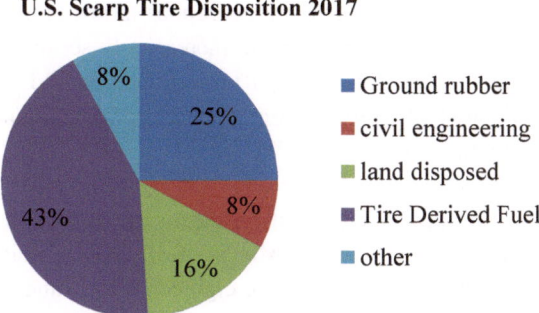

tire industry has prioritized the environmentally friendly and circular handling of waste tires. But the waste issue still exists. Due to their vast volume, waste tires are seen as an underappreciated resource worldwide and are a major environmental concern when disposed of in landfills. Rather than discarding waste materials following recycling, the use can make a big difference. Steel fiber extraction from used tires is becoming more and more popular. Utilizing waste recycled tire steel (WRTS) fibers which are derived from scrap tires in concrete present engineering application with the potential to be profitable. As per the U.S scarp tire disposition 2017 report (Fig. 4.3), it's clearly shows that only 8% of waste tires are using in the civil work and maximum are used for extracting the oil, but these process not suitable for our environment. However, there are still some difficulties to use of the waste tires.

Rubber leftovers were used as an insulating material for sound reduction as a result of the massive tire trash pile that resulted from the car revolution and a heightened environmental consciousness movement. A lot of studies have been conducted in recent years to create novel materials and technologies that improve sound absorption qualities. To minimize or reduce the high noise so many methods were introduced and among them the use of waste tire as insulation material is limited. In order to identify the study gaps for future studies in this area, this paper reviews the many aspects of waste tires, such as their mechanical, thermal, and sound-absorbing qualities. A summary and discussion of the available study findings and the tire recycling procedure are provided. Incorporating scrap tires as a sound-absorbing material is concluded to promote sustainable development by offering affordable, environmentally friendly, and mechanically superior building materials.

4.2   Literature Review

The number of tires removed from vehicles rises annually due to a significant increase in global in-vehicle demand brought on by the growing working population and the middle class's socioeconomic advancement. The disposal of waste tyre scraps poses a serious ecological risk because used rubber is not biodegradable. In recent years, the handling of trash tires has become an increasingly serious issue Glushankova et al. (2019). By the end of 2030, almost 1200 million tires would be wasted annually worldwide, with an estimated 112 million tires that are scrapped annually after being retread twice coming from India written by Wiśniewska et al. (2023). According to a recent World Health Organization (WHO) article (2018), traffic noise affects at least 100 million people in the European Union and results in the loss of at least 1.6 million years of healthy life annually. According to Mahan et al. (2019), noise pollution has been worse during the Industrial Revolution in the eighteenth and nineteenth centuries due to an increase in the use of machinery. The WHO report (1999), which addresses strategies for mitigating noise at the regional and local levels, notes that the problem's spread has been exacerbated by a number of other factors, such as an increase in road, rail, and aircraft traffic in addition to urbanisation and economic growth.

As per Yoon et al. (2006) Waste rubber is a durable material that negatively affects the ordinary natural environment despite its exceptional resistance to it. When a tire reaches the end of its useful life, a variety of management techniques are suggested for it, such as landfilling, re-treading and reuse, burning fuel, recycling to obtain raw materials, etc. Author Thomas et al. (2014) have to mention that used tires are disposed of in landfills, hazardous substances seep into the surrounding environment and cause major environmental issues. Because tires are impermeable, water may be kept in tire wastes for long periods, providing a breeding ground for rodents and mosquitoes. Aoudia et al. (2017) have written that the discarded tires take up a lot of space in stockpiles and landfills, which makes things harder because there isn't enough available land. Tire retreading is a cost-effective way to postpone the issue of disposal; but, as the tires reach the end of their useful lives, they are stacked up. The easiest and least expensive way to dispose of waste rubber tires is to burn them in the open. However, this method releases hazardous gases and volatile products into the atmosphere, including organic compounds, hydrocarbons, mercury, chromium, arsenic, cadmium, and others, which can cause serious fires and health risks mention by Epstein and Carhart (1953). Tire trash can be burned in designated furnaces or pyrolysis plants to recover energy. Tire waste can be recycled into crumb or shredded rubber, which can then be used in construction and other industries to reduce the waste's unwanted environmental impact observed by author Rowhani and Rainey (2016).

According to Oikonomou et al. (2007), there was a substantial build-up of tyre scrap following the automobile revolution and the rise in environmental consciousness. As a result, waste rubber materials were used in the construction sector beginning in the 1960s. Concrete and related building materials can be made from non-hazardous waste, which is primarily landfilled. The building industry plays a vital role in addressing the demands of urbanization and supports national economic expansion. As a result, professionals and researchers are enthusiastically developing new building technologies and employing recyclable waste materials to meet society's growing needs while adhering to stringent environmental laws. Authors Su et al. (2015) written as Waste rubber tires have been gradually substituting natural aggregate in concrete mixes and asphalt mixes in recent years to change the material's characteristics for less fatigue cracking, more durability, and lower cost observed by Kerekes et al. (2018). This has made it possible to dispose of scrap tires in a sustainable and economical manner.

A few works mainly address how rubber particles affect mechanical qualities, durability, workability, and density. On the other hand, while a synopsis of vibration damping, sound insulation, and thermal conductivity has been given, a thorough explanation of the methods employed for measurement has not. This chapter presents the fundamental characteristics of building materials for sustainable development and green building technology. It includes a summary of important features like thermal resistivity, acoustic material's ability to absorb sound, and a thorough explanation of the methods and techniques employed in the measurements. Following an extensive examination of the hybrid composites doped with recycled tire rubber in terms of thermal resistance, sound absorption, and vibration damping, the final section provides an overview of the practical uses of rubberized concrete for a range of purposes.

4.3   Materials and Methodology

As civilization has progressed, waste tire rubber has emerged as a significant waste material. This is because the need for vehicles is causing an increase in waste tire production at a faster pace. Therefore, techniques for recycling used tires must be developed. Many nations throughout the world are encouraging the recycling of old tires or the use of them as building materials in order to reduce environmental contamination. The issue of tyre disposal is being approached creatively in light of the current worldwide concern for the production of ecologically friendly products. These solutions include updating tyre life cycle evaluations, highlighting the advantages of recycling tyres, putting recovery plans in place, and figuring out how to turn waste tyres into resources that can be put to good use.

4.3.1   Recycling of Waste Tires

The chemical composition of tire rubber, fillers, and processing additives affects the mechanical properties and lifespan of car tires. Automobile tire recycling is especially difficult due to the vast range of composition elements and the poisonous nature of compounds. Crumb rubber can be made from discarded or scrap tyres before being put to use in various applications. Scrap tyres are made of textile, steel wire, and rubber. Tyres that are no longer needed must first be cut into smaller pieces in order to be used in another project. Tire processing is divided into two methods: mechanical and cryogenic.

Crumb rubber manufacture for the mechanical process entails shredding, chipping, and grinding of discarded tires into small sizes. Scrap tires are gathered by tire merchants and transported to the processing facility. Before use, the scrap tires are separated by size. A cracker mill or rotating corrugated steel drums are used to separate the steel wires from the sidewalls. Rubber shredding reduced rubber size from 100 to 50 mm. The size was then decreased from 50 to 10 mm in the first and second stages of the granulation process, according to Song et al. (2019). Steel fibre is removed using a screen and gravity separator. To make crumb rubber, tire chips are ground down to a smaller size.

After the steel wires have been extracted, tires are mechanically recycled (Fig. 4.4) by being broken up into small chips, scrap rubber, fine powder, and compounds of carbon for different applications.

According to the U.S tire Association the primary components of tire are natural fiber, textile, Steel, Synthetic Polymers, Fillers, and Antioxidants etc. In the below Fig. 4.5 the total percent of materials are mention.

To develop a set of polymer matrix composites, the current study uses a waste tire rubber crumb with a mesh size of 30 that was obtained from R. S. Rubber Industries, Khordha, as synthetic fibre reinforcement in an epoxy matrix. However, because waste tire has no mechanical strength on its own, it must be combined with a matrix material to form a solid structure. Understanding how to use epoxy to get rid of the rubber would help

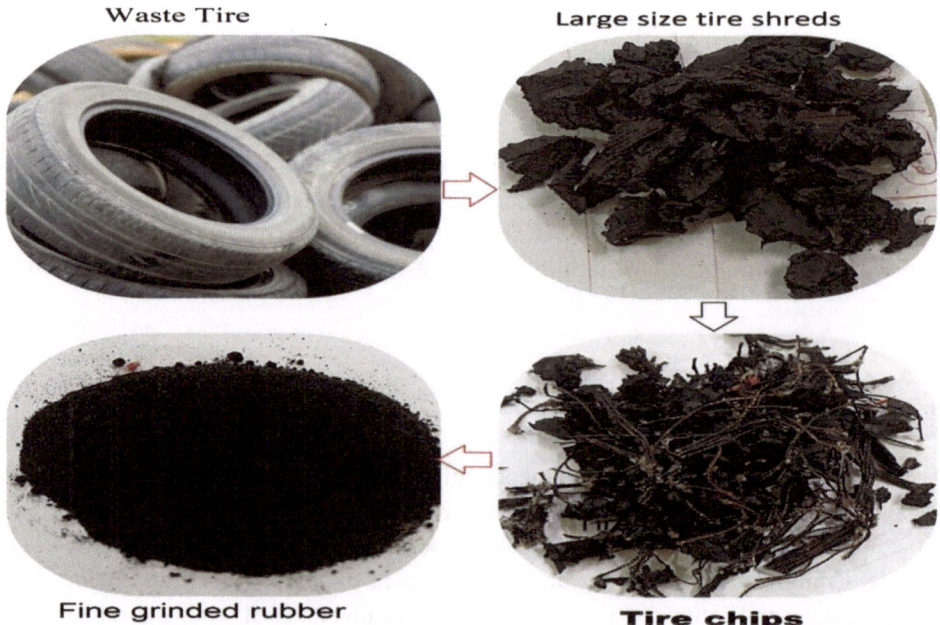

Fig. 4.4 Process of waste tire into fine rubber crumb

Fig. 4.5 Primary components percentage of car and Light trucks

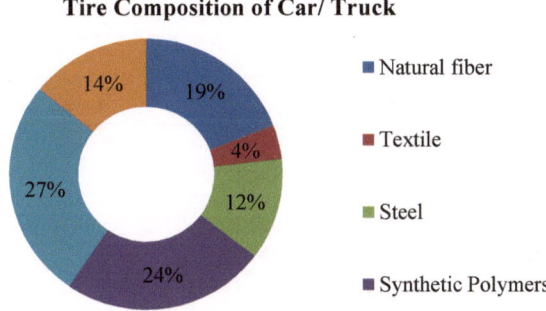

Tire Composition of Car/ Truck

- Natural fiber
- Textile
- Steel
- Synthetic Polymers

with the process of integrating the WTRC into more complex applications. Vulcanized rubber and other reinforcing materials are used to make tires. Synthetic rubber is the most widely used rubber matrix and is used for many different applications.

4.3.2   Epoxy Resin

The most commonly utilized polymers are polyester, epoxy, phenolic, polypropylene, and polyamide. Epoxy is a thermosetting resin that can undergo polymerization. Its many applications can be attributed to its high modulus, low creep, high tensile strength, minimal shrinkage, and superior corrosion resistance. However, the primary drawbacks of epoxy are its brittleness, length of drying time, and deterioration of characteristics when wet. Since epoxy has relatively low fracture energy, its toughness may be increased by using different rubbers. Because of their superior mechanical and electrical qualities, improved adherence to a broad range of fibres, and improved performance at higher temperatures, epoxy resins are the most widely used thermosetting polymers on the market for creating many advanced composites. They also exhibit low solidification-related shrinkage and strong chemical resistance. In the current study, epoxy (L-12) was used as the matrix material. Lapox L-12 is a medium viscosity liquid epoxy resin that is unchanged and can be used with different hardeners to create glass fibre-reinforced composites. The attributes that the cured composite must have and the processing technique to be employed determine which hardener to utilize. Hardener K-6 is a room temperature curing liquid hardener with low viscosity. For hand lay-up applications, it is frequently used. It has a short pot life and a quick cure at room temperature since it is fairly reactive. Operating temperatures exceeding 100 °C are possible for laminates. Table 4.1 describes the resin system's technical characteristics. The epoxy resin L-12 and hardener K-6 used in this investigation were provided by Herenba Instruments & Engineers Pvt. Ltd., Chennai.

Table 4.1 Technical properties of the resin system (Mashaan and Karim 2014)

Test (unit)	Typical values
Density of epoxy at 25 °C	1.1–1.2
Density of hardener at 25 °C	0.97–0.99
Tensile strength (MPa)	50–60
Hardness	70–80
Elastic modulus in tension (MPa)	4,400–4,600
Flexural strength (MPa)	130–150
Impact resistance (kj/m^2)	17–20
Water absorption (20 °C/10 days) (% w/w)	0.5–0.6
Compressive strength (N/mm^2)	110–120
Thermal conductivity (w/mK)	0.211

4.4 Methods

4.4.1 Composite Panel Manufacturing by Hand Layup Method

The hand-lay-up technique, a conventional and budget-friendly open molding method for composite production, was applied in this study to create the composites used. The epoxy resin (L12) and its hardener (K6) were mixed for 10 min at a 10:1 weight ratio, following the recommended procedure. The tire crumb was then added to the mixture, which was thoroughly mixed by hand. The Teflon paper was placed on the mould to facilitate removal and enhance the quality of the surface. To aid in removal, a silicon spray was applied to the mold's surface before pouring the epoxy-waste tyre mixture into the mould. After allowing the cured composite sample to cure for approximately 24 h, five specimens (Fig. 4.7) with a 15, 25, 35, 45, and 55% fibre weight fraction were produced and documented in Table 4.2.

Table 4.2 Designation of samples prepared

Designation	Weight fraction-based composition
Specimen-1(SP$_1$)	85% Epoxy + 15% WF of waste tire rubber crumb
Specimen-2(SP$_2$)	75% Epoxy + 25% WF of waste tire rubber crumb
Specimen-3(SP$_3$)	65% Epoxy + 35% WF of waste tire rubber crumb
Specimen-4(SP$_4$)	55% Epoxy + 45% WF of waste tire rubber crumb
Specimen-5(SP$_5$)	45% Epoxy + 55% WF of waste tire rubber crumb

This process has fewer conditions, and the manufacturing stages are straightforward. The general procedures used in this investigation to prepare epoxy-resin composites of different materials are listed in the attachment. Composite making is given step by step as follow.

- Collect the rubber crumb from the waste tire recycle company from Balasore, Odisha and put under the sun for removing the water particle.
- Combine the epoxy resin (L-12) and hardener (K-6) in a 10:1 ratio to create a combination that will yield material. After that fiber are added to this solution of epoxy resin and hardener in hand layup method.
- Next, two types of molds need to be made: a round mold whose diameter matches the impedance tube's diameter for sound testing, and a square mold for further mechanical and thermal testing needs.
- Add some realizing agent over the entire mold surface before pouring the liquid in. This will make it easier to remove the material from the mold once it has hardened.
- After that, all of the material was left for a full day under hydraulic pressure for a superior hardener. The material is taken out of the mold for inspection after the whole day has passed, and it is then put through a sound-absorbing test (Figs. 4.6 and 4.7).

4.5   Experimental Method

4.5.1   Sound Absorption Test

The evaluation of the sound absorption properties of the manufactured composite samples is carried out using the ASTM E1050-98 standard method, which involves the use of a medium-type impedance tube (see Fig. 4.8) equipped with two fixed microphones and a TestSens analyzing system. The impedance tube is used to measure various acoustical parameters within the frequency range of 500–5000 Hz. The sample to be tested is inserted into one end of the tube, while a loudspeaker is placed at the other end to serve as the sound source. The sound waves emitted from the loudspeaker enter the tube, strike the sample, and then bounce back. The sound pressure is monitored at two fixed locations using a two-channel digital frequency analyzer. The sound absorption coefficients (a) at different frequencies are then calculated by determining the complex transfer function. The value of the sound absorption coefficient ranges from 0 to 1, with 0 indicating complete sound rejection and 1 indicating complete sound absorption. Each sample has the same dimensions and shape as the cross-section of a round tube. The degree of sound absorption determines the sound absorption coefficient (α).

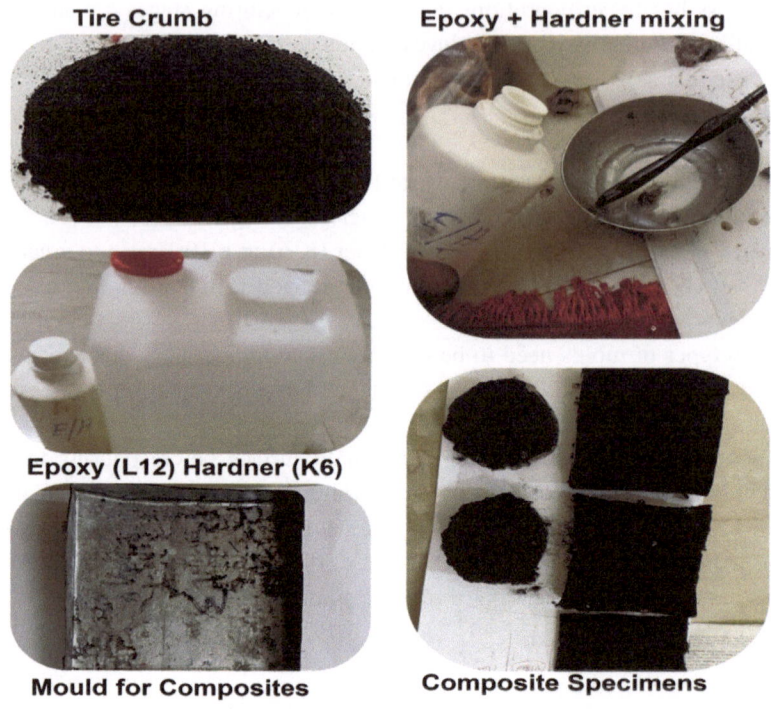

Fig. 4.6 Process of making composite material from the rubber crumb

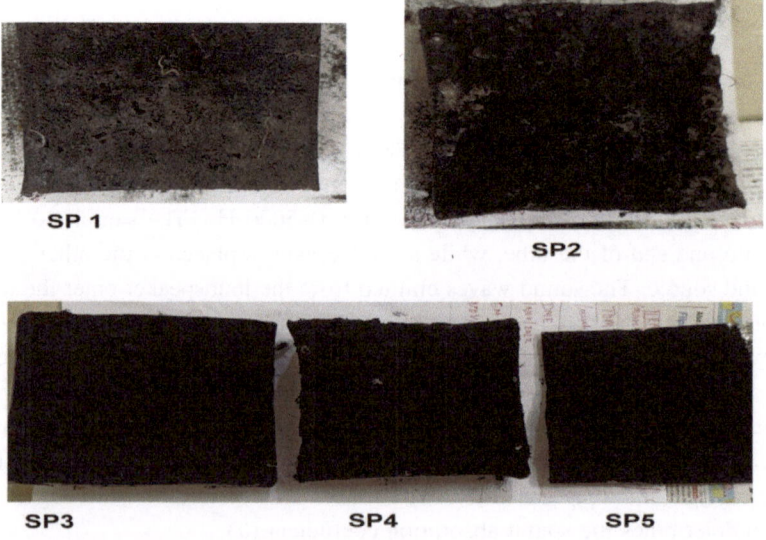

Fig. 4.7 Composite sample specimen of rubber crumb

Fig. 4.8 Block diagram of impedance tube

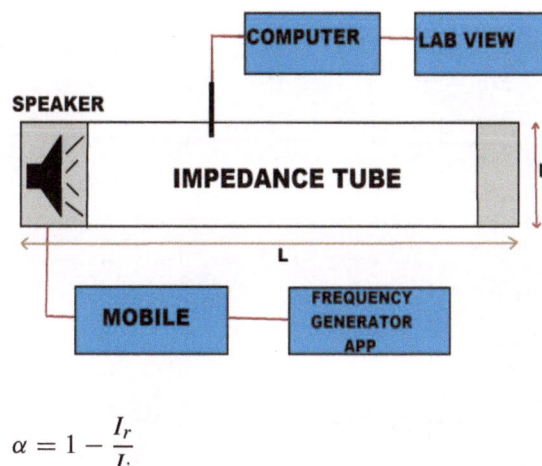

$$\alpha = 1 - \frac{I_r}{I_i}$$

where I_r = Reflected Sound Intensity

I_i = Incident Sound Intensity.

A material with a value of α more than 0.75 and a sound reflection value less than 0.25 are considered to be suitable options for sound absorption. The sound absorption coefficient was measured using three widely used techniques: the reverberation chamber, the reflection method, and the impedance tube. Because it is less expensive and simpler to evaluate, the impedance tube approach (Fig. 4.9) was utilized for sound absorption in this study.

4.5.2 Thermal Stability Test

The thermal conductivity of materials with varied warm conductivity, such as polymer, clay, elastic, composites, glass, and others, can be assessed using the thermal conductivity estimate device (Fig. 4.10). In the present experiment, this apparatus is used to measure the example's thermal conductivity at room temperature. ASTM E-1530 criteria are used to guide the analysis.

4.5.3 Tensile Test

In this study ASTM Standard D 638 (Fig. 4.11) was employed the tensile characteristics of the test specimens are assessed using a Universal Testing Machine of Fine Spavy Associates and Engineers Pvt. Ltd. (TUF- TUF - C 1000). The tests were run at a crosshead speed of 3 mm/min both before and after being exposed to moisture.. The specimens were

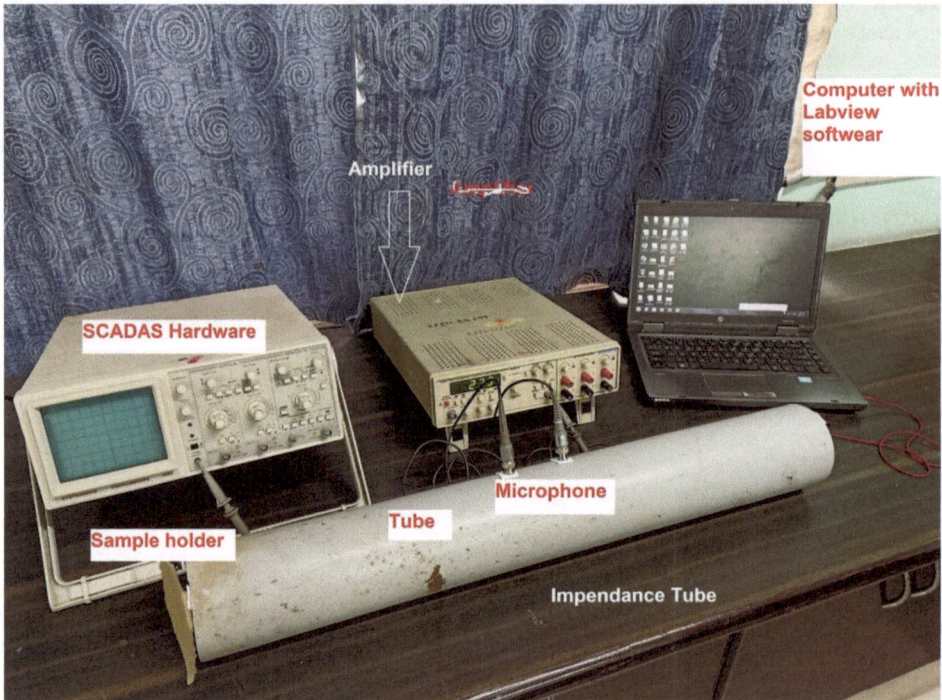

Fig. 4.9 Different parts of the impedance tube which are used in this experiment

carved into the shape of a dog bone using a micro-grinder. Five specimens were tested, and the average values were recorded throughout the test is the specimen's ultimate tensile strength, breaking strength, yield strength and percentage of elongation (tensile ductility) (Table 4.3).

4.5.4 Hardness Testing

A non-destructive hardness test measures a material's resistance to permanent deformation at its surface. It entails pressing a tougher material against the material under test. The Rockwell method measures hardness quickly and accurately on almost all metals and some polymers. It has a wide range of scales, making it useful for a variety of applications. In this experiment Zwick Roell (ASTM E 18 standard) hardness tester was used for measure the hardness of the specimen as shown in the Fig. 4.12.

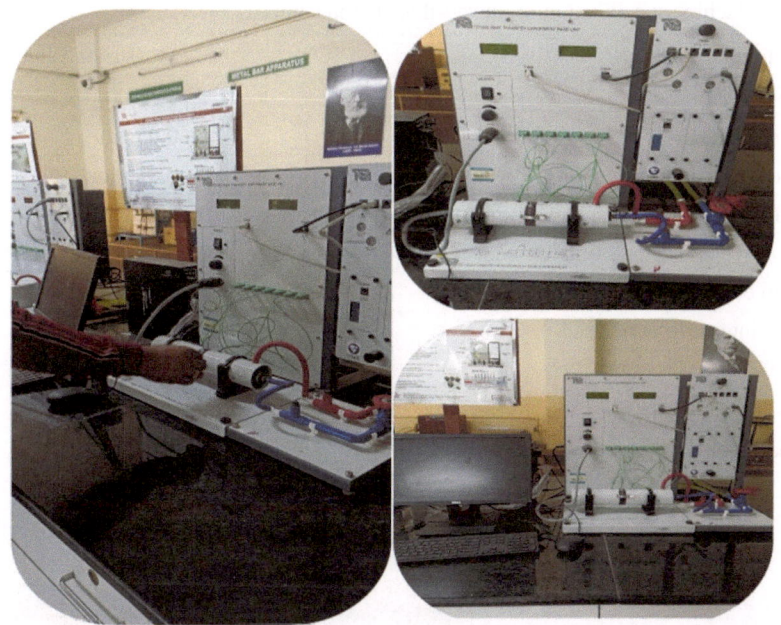

Fig. 4.10 Thermal conductivity testing machine

Fig. 4.11 Universal testing machines for tensile test of the specimen

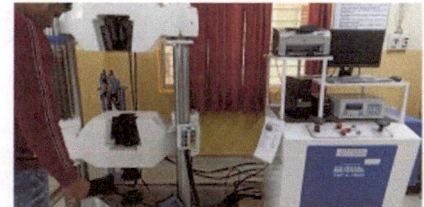

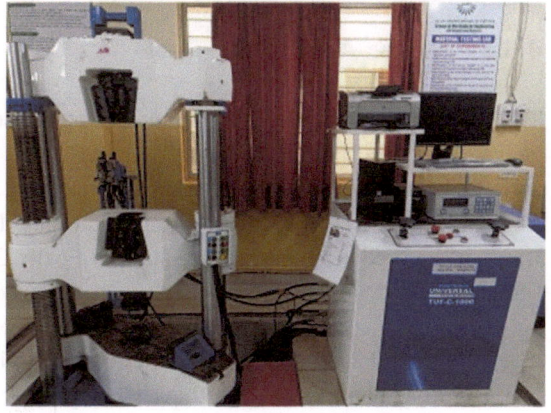

Table 4.3 Machine specification of universal testing machine

Specification	Measuring value
Measure capacity	0–1000 KN
Least count	0.05 KN
Resolution of piston movement	0.01 mm
Load range in KN with accuracy of measurement	20 1000
Max tensile clearance at a fully descended piston position	50–650 mm
Maximum clearance for compression test	0–650 mm
Max straining speed at no load	80 mm/min

Fig. 4.12 Rockwell hardness testing machine for measure hardness

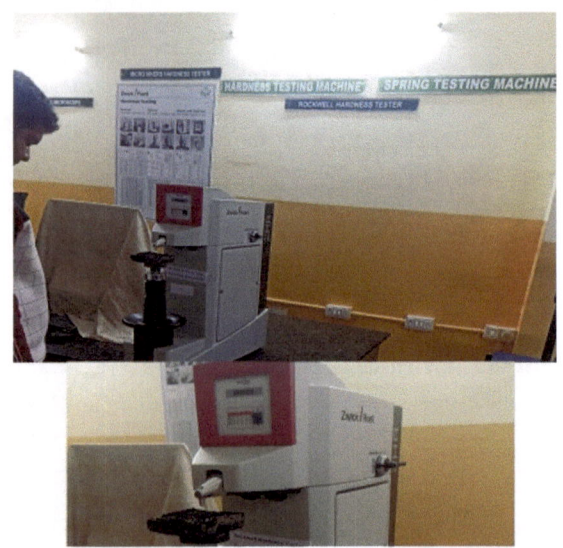

4.5.5   Water Absorption Test

The process of measuring the amount of water absorbed under particular circumstances is called water absorption. The specimens are dried in an oven at a predetermined temperature and time for the water absorption test, after which they are cooled in a desiccator. The specimens are weighed as soon as they cool. The substance is then submerged in water at the predetermined temperature typically 24 °C for a whole day or until equilibrium is reached. After being taken out of the specimen, it is dried with a lint-free cloth and weighed. The whole weight measurements were done by the Mettler Toledo balance. Mettler Toledo balances are excellent quality lab balances with check weighing, component counting, and other capabilities. They provide quick stabilization and response times as well as an accurate weigh/measurement display. The capacity of analytical balances

Fig. 4.13 Rubber crumb composite specimen immersed in the water for 24 h

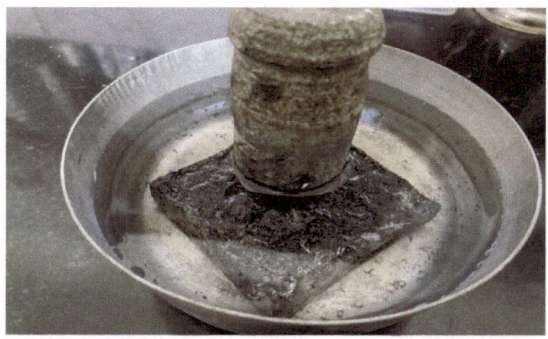

ranges from 5 to 520 g, and the readability ranges from 0.002 to 1 mg. The rubber crumb and epoxy composite specimen were immersed in the water by giving some external force for digging for 24 h, as shown in Fig. 4.13.

4.6 Results and Discussion

4.6.1 Water Absorption Test

For this studies Water absorption experiments were conducted by ASTM standards to investigate the water absorption property of the waste tire crumb-filled epoxy composites. A combination of composite samples was submerged for a while until saturation was reached in a deionized water bath at 24 °C. Before being cooled to room temperature, the samples were dried in an oven set at 50 °C for a whole day. After the specimen weight stabilized, the drying procedure was repeated. After 24 h, the test samples were taken out of the water and dried with a dry cloth then quickly weighed using a digital scale and a Mettler balance (Fig. 4.14) .

Percent Water Absorption $=$
$\left[(\text{Wet weight}(24\text{h in the water}) - \text{Dry weight}(\text{original weight}))/\text{Dry weight}\right] \times 100$

4.6.2 Tensile Test

All the specimen were tested in the above UTM (Universal testing machine) machine for find out the ultimate tensile strength, yield strength and Elongation (%) of that material and the values are shown in the below Table 4.4. The data indicate that tire crumb composite materials have much lower mechanical characteristics compared to the increase in epoxy, such as ultimate tensile strength. Furthermore, as the tire crumb weight percentage

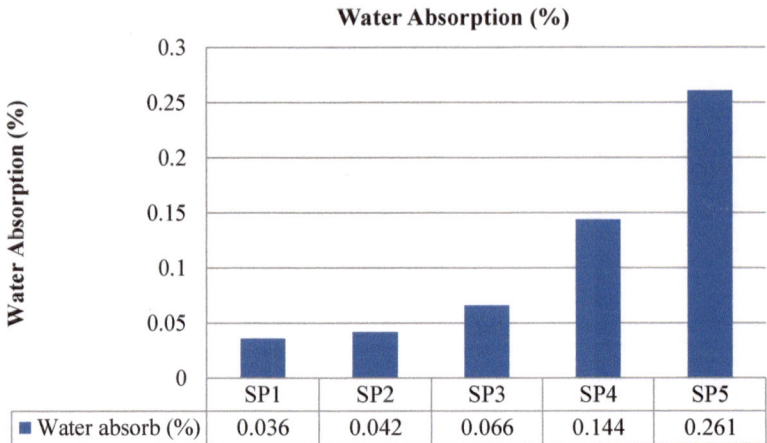

Fig. 4.14 Water absorption percentage by the specimen

increases, these mechanical qualities decrease. The primary causes of this degradation might be attributed to crumbed rubber's inferior mechanical qualities in comparison to epoxy and the weak bonding strength between the rubber surface and epoxy. This shows that as the tire crumb weight percentage rises inside the specimen's cross-section, the applied load magnifies the stresses and accelerates failure since the epoxy is primarily bearing the applied load.

Furthermore, as previously said, raising tire crumb weight fractions may cause an increase in tire crumb particle accumulations' porosity, voids, and spots, which might result in an uneven structure. During the production of the specimen, irregular mixing and pouring into the mould may be the cause of this non-uniformity (Sanjay et al., 2018) (Fig. 4.15 and Table 4.5).

Table 4.4 Samples' water absorption test results

No of specimen	Original weight (gm.)	Weight after 24h in water (gm.)	Change in weight (gm.)	Water absorb (%)
SP1	11.648	11.661	0.003	0.036
SP2	9.456	9.460	0.004	0.042
SP3	7.546	7.551	0.005	0.066
SP4	8.987	9.000	0.018	0.144
SP5	11.458	11.488	0.030	0.261

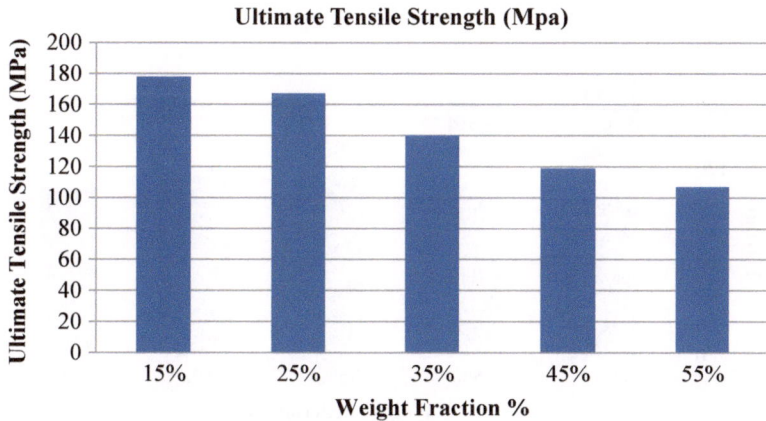

Fig. 4.15 Ultimate tensile strength versus tire crumb weight fraction

Table 4.5 Tensile test result of the composite specimen

Sample no	Yield strength (MPa)	Ultimate tensile strength (Mpa)	Elongation (%)
SP1	90	158	1.981
SP2	80	147	3.256
SP3	65	138	4.988
SP4	78	130	7.534
SP5	79	128	3.512

4.6.3   Hardness

Figure 4.16 illustrates how structural hardness changes as tire crumb weight fraction increases. It is evident that as the weight proportion of rubber material increases, the hardness decreases. The decreased hardness of crumbed rubber in comparison to the increased epoxy matrix may be the cause of this hardness drop. Furthermore, the cause for the decreasing structural strength with increased tire crumb might be the poor link between tire crumb and epoxy. Additionally, a rise in porosity and voids is typically linked to an increase in filler weight fraction, which has a detrimental influence on the hardness (Wiśniewska et al., 2023).

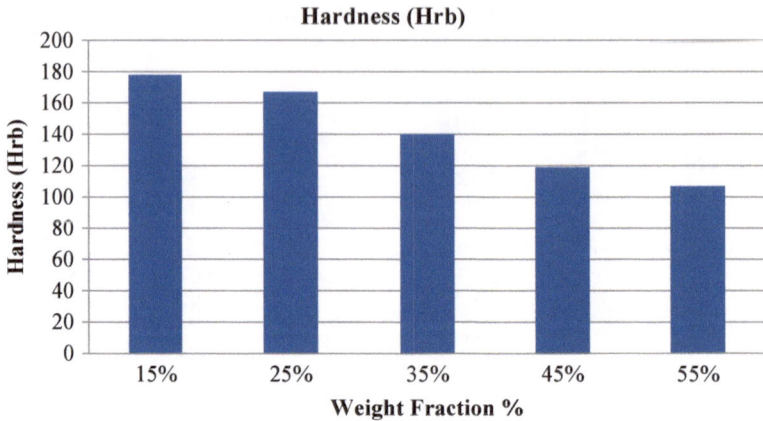

Fig. 4.16 Hardness versus tire crumb weight fraction

4.6.4 Density and Porosity

The Archimedes method, the sink-float method, or the density gradient method can all be employed to ascertain the composite density. This study utilizes the Archimedes principle to determine the actual density (ρa) of the composites. This procedure conforms to the standards set forth in ASTM D 792. The Archimedes principle posits that the apparent weight reduction of an object submerged in liquid is equal to the amount of liquid displaced by it (Table 4.6).

$$\text{Porosity} = 1 - (\text{Bulk density/Particledensity})$$

Table 4.6 Porosity result of rubber crumb composite

Specimen no	Thickness (in mm)	Experimental density (g/cm^3)	Theoretical density (g/cm^3)	Porosity (%)
SP1	5	1.10	1.120	1.785
SP2	8	1.04	1.086	4.235
SP3	10	0.99	1.043	5.081
SP4	13	0.95	1.027	7.497
SP5	15	0.92	1.000	8.000

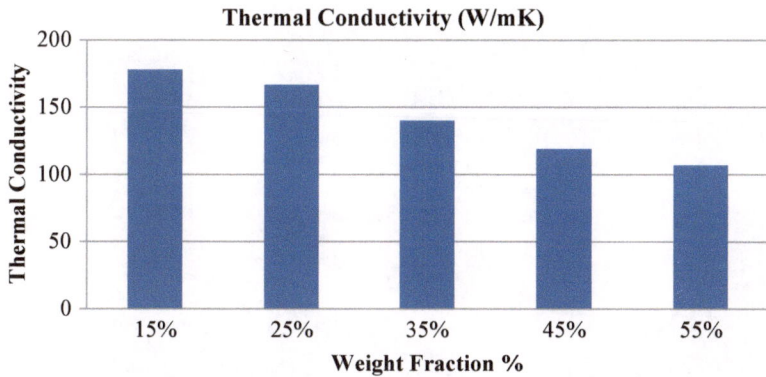

Fig. 4.17 Thermal Conductivity versus tire crumb weight fraction

4.6.5 Thermal Conductivity

Thermal conductivity was used to calculate the thermal insulation qualities of the samples. Figure 4.17 depicts the thermal conductivity of various samples. Low thermal conductivity numbers indicate more resistance to heat transmission through the material. Figure 4.17 shows the findings of testing on the heat conductivity of waste tire composites and epoxy. The thermal conductivity of composite materials is essentially determined by the thermal conductivity of the individual components, according to the mixing rule. Thermal conductivity increases with increasing temperature for all samples.

Furthermore, thermal conductivity may also be impacted by voids and porosity in the composite structure. The composite with a 15% waste tire volume percentage has less heat conductivity than the other samples, as can be seen in the results figure. This might be explained by the composite structure's high porosity, which is often linked to specimen preparation by hand lay-up. Additionally, it is evident that when the tire crumb percentage rises, the composite's thermal conductivity rises as well. Despite the poor heat conductivity of natural rubber, tire crumb may be efficiently made more thermally conductive by adding fibres and modification agents, especially carbon black (Sanjay et al., 2019).

4.6.6 Sound Absorption Coefficient Calculated with an Impedance Test Tube

Using an impedance tube, the sound absorption data were collected in the 500–5000 Hz frequency range (Fig. 4.18). The standard setup was utilized for all measurements conducted per ASTM E1050-10. To be more precise, the sound absorption coefficient (α) is used to assess the effectiveness of materials that absorb sound. The ratio of the initial

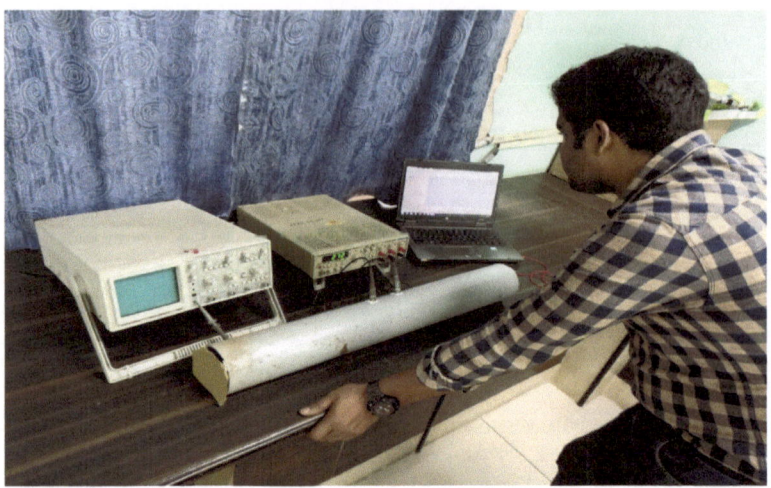

Fig. 4.18 Collect the SAC value of different composite material

(incident) and non-reflected (absorbed) sound intensities is known as the sound absorption coefficient. Complete reflection, or no sound absorption by the composites under test, is represented by a value between zero and one, while full absorption is represented by a value of one (Glushankova et al., 2019). Comparing composite materials to homogenous materials like pure metal, the latter have lower sound absorption coefficients. The fact comes about as a result of the cumulative effect of various acoustic energy losses. The sound wave interacts with several types of suspended particles across the inhomogeneous mediums that are different from the matrix in terms of density, compressibility, and thermo physical properties. Consequently, there are greater losses of acoustic energy than there are in the matrix (Table 4.7).

The noise reduction coefficient can be defined as the average of all the sound absorption coefficients measured at various frequencies. Finding a specimen's maximal capacity to absorb sound is simple once we have the noise reduction coefficient.

Noise Reduction Coefficient (NRC)

$$\alpha = \frac{\alpha_{500} + \alpha_{1000} + \alpha_{1500} + \alpha_{2000} + \alpha_{2500} + \alpha_{3000} + \alpha_{3500} + \alpha_{4000} + \alpha_{4500} + \alpha_{5000}}{10}$$

Perfect absorption is indicated by an NRC of 1, whilst idealized reflection is shown by an NRC of 0. So from the above table it is clearly shows that the composites containing 15% weight of waste tire crumb exhibited comparatively low sound absorption. With a noise reduction value of 0.341, the sound coefficient (α) values vary from 0.213 to 0.451 when the frequencies are changed. However, an increase in tyre crumb content might lead to an increase in the sound absorption coefficient, especially at higher concentrations. In

Table 4.7 Noise reduction coefficient (NRC) of specimens

Frequency (in Hz)	SP1	SP2	SP3	SP4	SP5
500	0.213	0.221	0.406	0.641	0.745
1000	0.326	0.351	0.751	0.784	0.799
1500	0.354	0.507	0.657	0.599	0.721
2000	0.259	0.501	0.459	0.716	0.612
2500	0.395	0.557	0.454	0.728	0.846
3000	0.421	0.498	0.759	0.643	0.761
3500	0.254	0.314	0.637	0.642	0.799
4000	0.326	0.474	0.326	0.604	0.748
4500	0.412	0.521	0.72	0.771	0.809
5000	0.451	0.572	0.673	0.732	0.884
(NRC)	0.341	0.452	0.584	0.686	0.772

the higher side of composites containing 55% weight of waste tire crumb shows the value varies from 0.745 to 0.884 with the noise reduction coefficient vale of 0.772, which also a good absorbing ability.

As the material thickness grows, so do the sound absorption qualities, as seen in Fig. 4.19. In the experiment, Specimen 1 had a lower thickness value, i.e., 5 mm, so the sound absorption value was also very poor, i.e., 0.341. That means the value of thickness is directly proportional to the sound absorbing capacity of a material in case acoustic material.

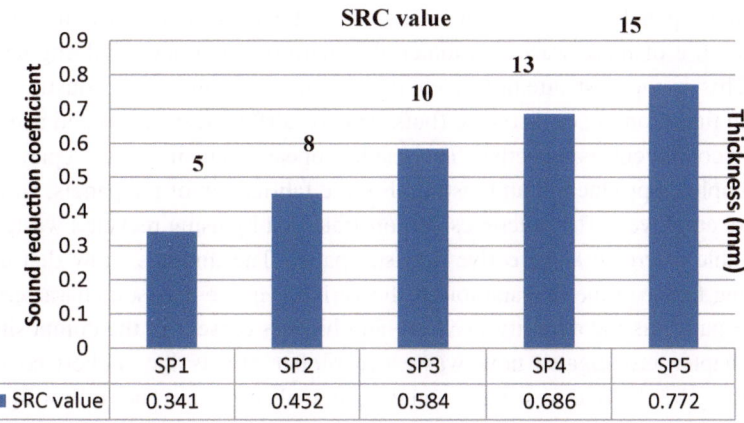

Fig. 4.19 Graph between sound absorption coefficients versus thickness

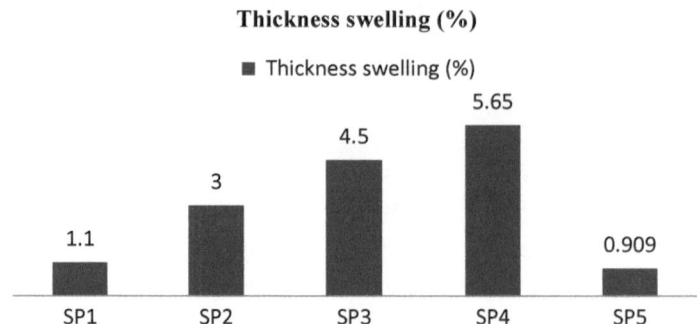

Fig. 4.20 Thickness swelling of test sample specimen

4.6.7 Thickness Swelling

The samples' thickness swelling (TS) were assessed in accordance with ASTM D1037 guidelines. The samples were left at room temperature for a full day while submerged horizontally. The samples were emptied of extra water and their thickness was measured after each submersion interval (Fig. 4.20).

4.7 Conclusion

Waste tire disposal will remain a global challenge as long as waste tire collection keeps increasing. The ideal and sustainable way to prevent its detrimental effects on the environment is to use recycled tire waste rubber as a sound-absorbing substance. Using wasted tires to make panels with good acoustic characteristics is an intriguing technique to prolong the life of these wastes in materials, environmental, and civil engineering applications. This is the first attempt at characterizing the composite acoustic panels made from scrap tires from a non-acoustic (bulk density, airflow resistance) and acoustic (sound absorption coefficient) perspective. The results appear promising. Five separate composite panels completed production and testing. For the fabrication of the panels, various mixing ratios were employed. The outcomes demonstrate that by using recycled waste tire crumb, we were able to create an effective acoustic panel. The findings show that a significant contributing factor to the explanation of the variance in the acoustic characteristics of the composite panels is the quantity of waste and binders present in the composite material.

   This chapter investigates how waste tire rubber affects the rubberized composite's tensile strength, thermal resistance, and sound absorption. The following significant conclusions are reached.

From spent crumbed tire rubber, an affordable, ecologically friendly composite with suitable mechanical qualities can be created. The recycled tire rubber's size and texture have a significant effect on the performance of composite materials. For this reason, old tires are recycled using several grinding techniques into a range of sizes, including chipped, crumb, and finely ground rubber. As the sound absorption property of the material increases due to the increase in porosity and air flow resistance, different shapes and sizes of waste tire pieces are required.

The decrease in sound wave amplitude that occurs when a sound wave passes through a medium is known as sound absorption. Rubberized composites have larger porosity, which causes more sound waves to scatter and significantly reduces the amplitude of the sound waves that are transmitted. As a result, as rubber content rises, so does the noise reduction coefficient, with sound absorption becoming more noticeable at frequencies higher than 500 Hz. From the Table-5 it is clearly shows that increase the thickness and porosity that increases the SAC value of a material. Statistical, experimental studies revealed that samples with 15% tire crumb had the highest thermal conductivity and that this value declined as the proportion of tires increased. However, samples with high epoxy had lower thermal conductivity because of their lower porosity. Waste tire crumb can be used as an epoxy matrix as a filler material to improve sound insulation and boost heat conductivity but at the expense of mechanical strength.

The results show that, in proportion to the percentage increase in waste tire rubber crumb combinations and decrease hardness, and tensile strength. Therefore, in order to improve the mechanical qualities, more glue must be added. Form the above experiment it also showed that increase the thickness of the composite material must affect the sound absorption coefficient. If the material has more thickness and porosity it absorbs more sound. So in this experiment it also shows that the waste tire can be used as a sound insulator for the different noisy environment. The result shows a good result that can be used in home appliances where sound is quite unpleasant, like a mixture grinder, washing machine sound, or vacuum cleaner during operation.

References

Abdulhameed, J. I., Ali, A. H., & Kara, I. H. (2022, December). Developing crumbed rubber tires/epoxy composite, by surface treatment with different silane coupling agents. In *Materials science forum* (Vol. 1077, pp. 39–45). Trans Tech Publications Ltd.

Aoudia, K., Azem, S., Hocine, N. A., Gratton, M., Pettarin, V., & Seghar, S. (2017). Recycling of waste tire rubber: Microwave devulcanization and incorporation in a thermoset resin. *Waste Management, 60*, 471–481.

Epstein, P. S., & Carhart, R. R. (1953). The absorption of sound in suspensions and emulsions. I. Water fog in air. *The Journal of the Acoustical Society of America, 25*(3), 553–565.

Glushankova, I., Ketov, A., Krasnovskikh, M., Rudakova, L., & Vaisman, I. (2019). End of life tires as a possible source of toxic substances emission in the process of combustion *8*(2), 113

Kerekes, Z., Lubloy, E., & Kopecsko, K. (2018). Behaviour of tyres in fire. *Journal of Thermal Analysis and Calorimetry*. https://doi.org/10.1007/s10973-018-7001-9

Khaloo, A. R., Dehestani, M., & Rahmatabadi, P. (2008). Mechanical properties of concrete containing a high volume of tire–rubber particles. *Waste Management, 28*(12), 2472–2482.

Mahan, H. M., Farhan, M. M., & Shaalan, T. G. (2019). Studying some mechanical properties of river shell particle polymer matrix composite. *Journal of Southwest Jiaotong University, 54*(4), 1–7.

Mashaan, N. S., & Karim, M. R. (2014). Waste tyre rubber in asphalt pavement modification. *Materials Research Innovations, 8*. https://doi.org/10.1179/1432891714Z.000000000922

Murgel, E. (2007). *Fundamentos de Acústica Ambiental*. São Paulo, Brazil: Senac. https://atlantisfiber.com/tires-recycling-and-taking-them-off-the-road/

Rowhani, A., & Rainey, T. J. (2016). Scrap tyre management pathways and their use as a fuel—A review. *Energies, 9*(11), 1–26.

Sanjay, M. R., Madhu, P., Jawaid, M., et al. (2018). Characterization and properties of natural fiber polymer composites: A comprehensive review. *Journal of Cleaner Production, 172*, 566–581.

Sanjay, M. R., Siengchin, S., Parameswaranpillai, J., et al. (2019). A comprehensive review of techniques for natural fibers as reinforcement in composites: Preparation, processing and characterization. *Carbohydrate Polymers, 207*, 108–121.

Song, J.-P., Tian, K.-Y., Ma, L.-X., Li, W., & Yao, S.-C. (2019). The effect of carbon black morphology to the thermal conductivity of natural rubber composites. *International Journal of Heat and Mass Transfer, 137*, 184–191.

Su, H., Yang, J., Ghataora, G.S., & Dirar, S. (2015). Surface modified used rubber tyre aggregates: Effect on recycled concrete performance. *Magazine of Concrete Research, 67*(12), 680–691. https://www.goldsteinresearch.com/report/global-tire-recycling-industry-market-trends-analysis#:~:text=Every%20year%20over%201.6%20billion,100%20million%20tires%20every%20year, https://5.imimg.com/data5/VR/WS/MY-34403803/lapox-epoxy-resin-l12-with-hardener-k-6-1-1-kg-packing.pdf, https://datatopics.worldbank.org/what-a-waste/trends_in_solid_waste_management.html

Thomas, B. S., Gupta, R. C., Kalla, P., & Cseteneyi, L. (2014). Strength, abrasion and permeation characteristics of cement concrete containing discarded rubber fine aggregates. *Construction and Building Materials, 59*, 204–212.

Wiśniewska, P., Haponiuk, J. T., Colom, X., & Saeb, M. R. (2023). Green approaches in rubber recycling technologies: Present status and future perspective. *ACS Sustainable Chemistry & Engineering*.

World Health Organization—WHO. (1999). *Guidelines for community noise*.

World Health Organization—WHO. (2018). *Environmental Noise guidelines for the European region* (p. 160).

Yoon, S., Prezzi, M., Siddiki, N. Z., & Kim, B. (2006). Construction of a test embankment using a sand–tire shred mixture as fill material. *Waste Management, 26*, 1033–1044.

Home Appliance Noise Reduction with a Composite Made of Waste Tire Crumb and Epoxy Resin: A Case Study

5

5.1 Introduction

According to Jariwala et al. (2017), excessive noise and vibration diminish lifespans and lead to structural failures. Government regulations designed to reduce noise pollution in society demonstrate the importance of the noise problem. The main sources of noise generation, sometimes known as "noise pollution," include air and surface traffic, industrial machines, home appliances, and construction activities. In addition to being annoying, noise pollution poses a health danger to nearby residents. According to Raj et al. (2020), noise can be heard everywhere there is life, including in forests, offices, homes, and even underwater. The World Health Organization states that human hearing can tolerate noise levels up to 70dB. The use of household appliances has increased dramatically in recent years, and the noise pollution that produces is a serious threat to public health in home environments. Noise pollution harms human existence; it is irritating, interferes with speech and sleep, and lowers productivity at work (Mohanty & Fatima, 2015a, 2015b).

Asdrubali et al. (2012) have been written the variety and frequency of use of home facilities and appliances in residential areas have increased as living standards have increased. Refrigerators, washing machines, vacuum cleaners, mixer grinders, and kitchen utensils are examples of indoor equipment that have an open layout and significantly affect the noise level of nearby interior spaces. From the viewpoint of home designers, additional efforts ought to be made to improve the noise environment and regulate the interior equipment's source level. Soundproofing materials, which work well as dampers, barriers, and absorbers in household appliances, can help solve these issues (Thilagayathi et al., 2010). The effect that consumable items have on the environment is another crucial factor that needs to be taken into account. Recent writers have acknowledged and executed the significance of using waste materials in potential domains of application. Not

© The Author(s), under exclusive license to Springer Nature Switzerland AG 2025
S. Satapathy et al., *Noise Pollution and Ergonomic Intervention by Acoustic Material*,
Synthesis Lectures on Mechanical Engineering,
https://doi.org/10.1007/978-3-031-66308-6_5

enough work has gone into this, and no plan has been presented to deal with the problems or the condition of noisy indoor equipment in households as of yet.

5.2 Noise Control Materials

According to Crocker (1981), the aircraft industry has mostly depended on technology based on synthetic fibre composites made of carbon, glass, or Kevlar since 1950 in order to reduce noise. After meeting aircraft criteria, developments in composite design are aimed at the home and general industrial sectors. In contrast, noise pollution has become an issue due to the growing use of mechanical and electrical appliances in business and at home. Despite having unique qualities like as rigidity, high strength-to-weight ratio, and low weight, synthetic composites are not well suited for use in the home and industrial sectors because of the expensive cost of the raw ingredients. Another waste which is pliantly available in the environment is waste tire. As per the report by the end of 2030, almost 1200 million tires would be wasted annually worldwide, with an estimated 112 million tires that are scrapped annually 'after being retread twice coming from India. So in this study waste tire was used for alternative of other type of insulation material, as the waste tire is pliantly available, less cost and recyclables.

5.2.1 Manufacturing and Properties of Waste Tire Crumb

Waste tires are one of the many waste materials that have accumulated on Earth. Tires have a short lifespan and are in high demand, leading to a rising amount of garbage. Therefore, it's crucial to create techniques for recycling waste tires. Because of its important attributes, which include being affordable, recyclable, and availability on the environmentally, research on waste tire crumb reinforced composites is advancing rapidly. In this research Waste tires were used as reinforcing material. Rubber crumbs are created from vehicle trash tires. These can be created using a variety of mechanical processes as well as cryogenics. The specimen was prepared using the hand lay-up method, which is one of the easiest. The technique requires minimal resources and is straightforward. For the first time, an attempt has been made to characterize the composite acoustic panels manufactured from scrap tires from both an acoustic (sound absorption coefficient) and non-acoustic (bulk density, airflow resistance) standpoint. The findings seem encouraging. The results indicate that the amount of waste and binders in the composite material has a major role in explaining the variation in the acoustic properties of the composite panels.

5.2.2   Noise Control by Home Appliances

Advancements in technology have led to the compact and efficient design of household appliances, including washing machines, dryers, refrigerators, and vacuum cleaners, which are commonly seen in residential structures. The use of household appliances has increased noise pollution those produce is a serious threat to public health in residential settings. It was chosen to utilize Waste tire crumb felt for sound absorption based on the results of the flammability and acoustical tests conducted on the tire crumb and epoxy resin composite samples. All five of the hypothetical radiating surfaces had their sound intensities mapped in order to determine the sources of noise in the household appliance. Following the identification and ranking of the noise sources, the suitable noise control was determined by absorbing and applying the created tire crumb composite. After tire crumb treatment, the appliance's temperature does not noticeably alter.

5.3   Literature Review

When it comes to techniques for measuring noise, Tandon et al. (1997) ranked and analysed the sources by measuring the sound intensity of a two-wheeler scooter's engine. Sound intensity, not sound pressure, was used to determine sound power during testing, even though a constant background noise level could be tolerated. Two microphones were used in a sound intensity technique to measure and locate the source of the noise. Crocker (1981) experimented to assess the noise level and sound intensity of a residential split system air conditioner using a two-microphone sound intensity probe. Pilot tests on washing machine, vacuum cleaner and mixture grinder are carried out in an effort to determine whether produced jute goods may be used to reduce household appliance noise. Our research on a few modern home appliances provided fresh insight into the value and potential uses of these materials for noise control across a wide range of sectors.

5.4   Methodology

It was determined to employ tyre crumb for sound absorption based on the results of the acoustical and thermal testing of the waste tyre crumb samples in the preceding chapter. The sound intensities of each of the five potential radiating surfaces were mapped in order to identify the sources of noise in the home appliance. The SIL measurements were carried out by a B&K 2260 Investigator system using a sound intensity probe. Following the identification and ranking of the noise sources, the appropriate noise control was determined by absorbing and applying the created tire composite. After being treated with tire, the appliance's temperature does not significantly change.

Fig. 5.1 Vacuum cleaner

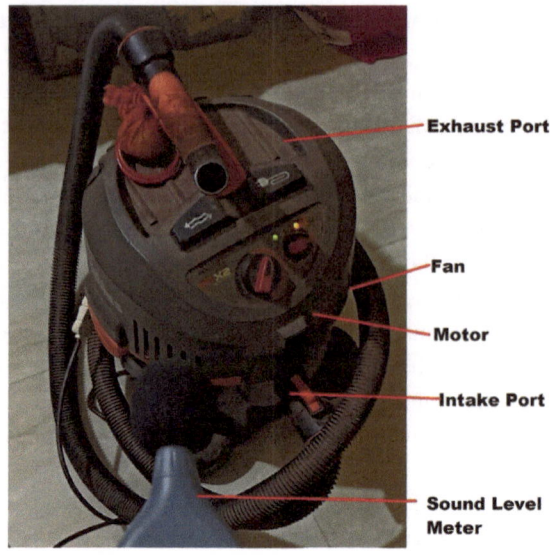

5.4.1   Case Study-1 Vacuum Cleaner

The experiment was conducted using a Eureka Forbes Euro vacuum cleaner, as seen in Fig. 5.1. This dryer weighs 6.67 kg and has the following measurements: 330 × 355 × 490 mm. The motor's suction and blower capacities are 22.55 KPA and 1400 l/min, respectively. It also as has sounds level of 85 dB. Using point measuring technique and sound intensity mapping, the vacuum cleaner's noise source was identified. After finding the noise source, measure the sound level on four different sides without using a sample. After collecting the data, put the sample on the five sides of the vacuum cleaner and collect the data.

5.4.2   Case Study-2 Washing Machine

For this case study, a BOSCH Industries washing machine was utilized as shown in the below Fig. 5.2. The washing machine weighs 26 kg and measures 530 × 600 × 720 mm in its physical dimensions. The ratings for the heater and motor are 1.8 kW and 300 W, respectively. This machine can clean up to 7 kg of wet clothes in a single operation cycle. Every experiment was carried out in both empty and loaded condition. Using point measuring technique and sound intensity mapping, the washing machine's noise source was identified. After finding the noise source, measure the sound level on four different sides without using a sample. After collecting the data, put the sample on the four sides of the washing machine and collect the data.

Fig. 5.2 Washing machine

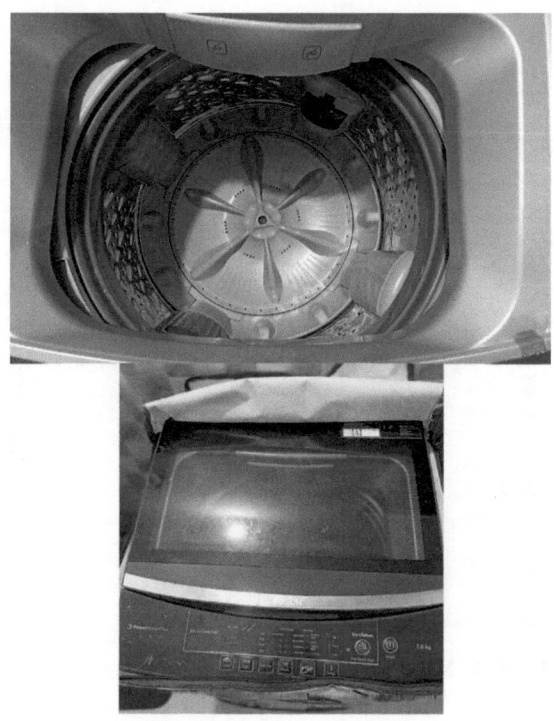

5.4.3   Case Study-3 Mixer Grinder

For this case study, a Sumeet company mixer grinder was utilized with the physical dimension of 28.3D × 20W × 29.5H Centimeters, 1500 W power, and 3.5 kg weight as shown in the Fig. 5.3. Each experiment was run with both a loaded and an empty condition. The source of the noise coming from the washing machine was located using sound intensity mapping and point measuring technique. Measure the sound pressure level four times on separate sides without using a sample after locating the source of the noise. Place the sample on all four sides of the mixer grinder and continue collecting data after that.

5.5   Result Discussion

5.5.1   Case Study-1 Vacuum Cleaner

An acoustical measurement technique was used to apply the vacuum cleaner's noise control. Tyre crumb was also used as a sound-absorbing substance in this case study. The entire trial was carried out under both loading and unloading circumstances (Table 5.1).

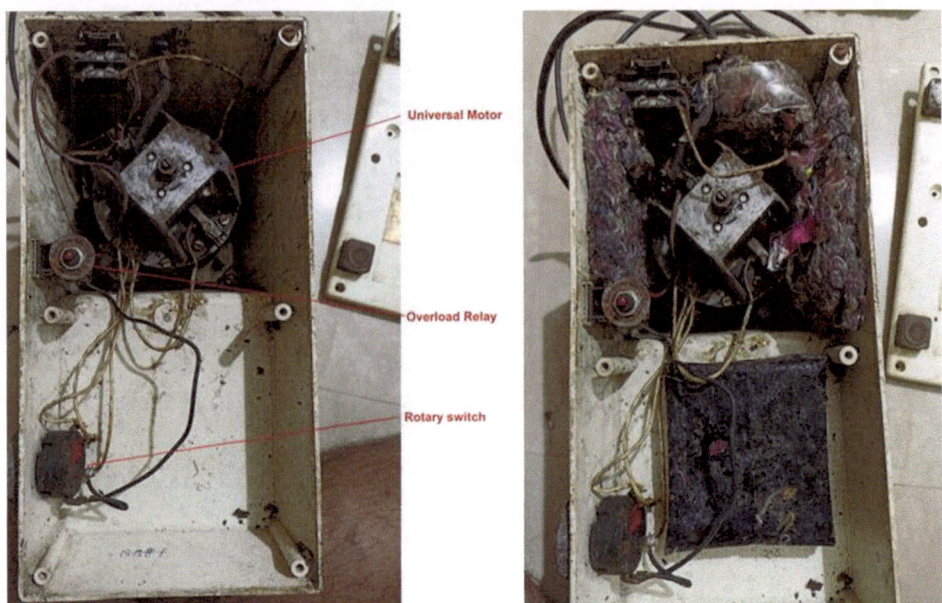

Fig. 5.3 Mixer grinder

Table 5.1 Average sound pressure levels at each of the vacuum cleaner's surrounding faces both with and without acoustical treatment

Surface	Without treatment (SWL) dB	With treatment (SWL) dB	Difference dB
Right	95.4	85.8	9.6
Left	94.3	85.4	8.9
Front	95.3	87.3	8
Back	94.2	85.2	9
Top	97.1	88.2	8.9

5.5.2 Case Study-1 Washing Machine

The washing machine's noise control system used an analogous acoustical measurement technique. This case study also used tire crumb composite as a sound-absorbing material. The whole experiment was conduct on both loading and unloading condition. For getting the best result take the two value of each condition (without treatment and with treatment). Table 5.2 lists the average sound power at each surrounding face of the home dryer, both with and without an acoustical blanket. Due to the placement of the motor and blower, the back (rear) surface is the one that radiates the most when the dryer surfaces are not treated. The Table 5.3 illustrates that the back side of the washing machine that produces the most

Table 5.2 Average sound pressure levels at each of the vacuum cleaner's surrounding faces both with and without acoustical treatment

Surface	Without treatment (SWL) dB	With treatment (SWL) dB	Difference dB
Right	78.2	75.3	2.9
Left	77.3	74.3	3
Front	67.2	64.2	3
Back	78.1	75.3	3.1

Table 5.3 Average sound pressure levels at each of the Mixer Grinder's surrounding faces both with and without acoustical treatment

Surface	Without treatment (SWL) dB	With treatment (SWL) dB	Difference dB
Right	85.2	79.1	6.1
Left	84.2	79.2	5
Front	84.2	79.2	5
Back	84.1	79.1	5
Bottom	87.8	80.1	7.7

sound. Since the dryer's motor and fan are located on its back side, an experiment was carried out to determine the sound level at the bottom level. Without treatment, the sound level was 75.3 dB, and with treatment, it was 78.1 dB. The specimen was pasted on all sides of the washing machine. Thus, the sound level dropped to 3.1 dB following therapy. Thus, the application of sound-absorbing material yields certain noteworthy outcomes.

5.5.3 Case Study-1 Mixer Grinder

The noise management of the mixer grinder was implemented using an acoustical measurement approach of the same kind as in cases 1 and 2. In this case study, tyre crumb was also utilized as a sound-absorbing material. The whole experiment was conducted in both loading and unloading conditions. For the best result, take the two values of each condition (without treatment and with treatment).

In the below table, it shows that the maximum sound is produced from the bottom side of the mixture. Because the motor and fan are both situated on the bottom side of the grinder, after pasting the entire specimen on all sides of the mixer wall, the experiment was conducted, and that shows that at the bottom level, without treatment, the sound level was 87.8 dB, and with treatment, it was 80.1 dB. So after treatment, the sound level decreased to 7.7 dB. Hence, the use of sound-absorbing material shows some significant results.

5.6   Conclusion

According to the results of the previously mentioned case studies, the waste tire offers a lot of promise for use in noise reduction applications. An alternative to the conventional synthetic fibers used for noise reduction is waste tire. Analyses of the sound intensity on a vacuum cleaner, mixing grinder, and washing machine were made to pinpoint the noise's origin. The vacuum cleaners sound output level was lowered by 10 dB by employing a closed enclosure lined with waste tire composite material. After applying a waste tire composite, the dryer's emitted sound power level was reduced by an overall 6 dB and in case of grinder the sound level reduced to 10 dB by employing the composite specimen. It has been discovered that composites made of tire crumb have great thermal stability, high porosity, high sound absorbing capacity, and medium thermal insulation. This study suggests using tire crumb and epoxy composites, (a lightweight, recyclable, and easily available material) to reduce noise in household appliances. In light of these positive findings, it is suggested that waste tire be utilized as a noise-reducing material for home appliances, such as the dishwasher, refrigerator, Air conditioner and hair dryer etc.

References

Asdrubali, F., Schiavoni, S., & Horoshenkov, K. V. (2012). A review of sustainable materials for acoustic applications. *Building Acoustics, 19*(4), 283–312. https://doi.org/10.1260/1351-010X.19.4.283

Crocker, M. J. (1981). The use of existing and advanced intensity techniques to identify noise sources on a diesel engine. *SAE Transactions*, 2227–2238.

Jariwala, H. J., Syed, H. S., Pandya, M. J., & Gajera, Y. M. (2017). Noise pollution & human health: A review. *Noise and Air Pollutions: Challenges and Opportunities, Ahmedabad: LD College of Eng*

Mohanty, A. R., & Fatima, S. (2015a). Noise control using green materials. *Sound & Vibration, 49*, 13–15.

Mohanty, A. R., & Fatima, S. (2015b). Biocomposites for industrial noise control. In V. K. Thakur & M. R. Kessler (Eds.), *Green biorenewable biocomposites from knowledge to industrial applications* (pp. 220–261). Apple Academic Press.

Raj, M., Fatima, S., & Tandon, N. (2020). Recycled materials as a potential sound absorbers: A study on denim shoddy and waste jute fibers. *Applied Acoustics, 159*, 107070.

Tandon, N., Nakra, B. C., Sarkar, B., & Adyanthaya, V. (1997). Noise control of two-wheeler scooter engine. *Applied Acoustics, 51*(4), 369–380.

Conclusion and Ergonomics Study of Residential Facing Noise Issue

6.1 Ergonomics Study of Residential Facing Noise Issue

Noise not only hampers listening capacity, also impacts on mental health. Discomfort of mental health affects both physical health (cardiac arrest, nerve problems, head ache etc.) and psychological effects (behavioral changes, accidents, mental issues).Hence to studying ergonomic mental well ness and impact of noise on human health.

To study and analyse the effects of residential noise on human health, a small study is carried on to study on psychological stress level due to noise. Hence, Ergonomic architectural analysis is conducted and designs suggested helping avoid noise pollution and its adverse effect on human health. Table 6.1 Noise measurements before and after use of Acoustic material in a 12 by 12 drawing room with door and window closed. It shows that the noise is drastically reduced inside a room as well as outside the room. Hence, use of acoustic materials will provide a better solution and protect human health. Table 6.2 shows the shape and size of acoustics based on maximum noise absorbing capacity. It was found that compared to other shapes of the acoustic membrane after placing the plane, acoustic material maximum noise is absorbed. Table 6.3 shows average perception of residential after using noise absorbing material in Likert scale (0 = no, 1 = yes). 50 Indian customers have given their perception, when they were allowed to spend 7–8 h in a room for 3–4 days where acoustic materials, particularly waste tyres were used. It was found that a maximum of 45 people have discomfort level decreases after use of acoustic material in their room. Table 6.4 shows Economic Analysis of Acoustic materials and the cost found was Rs. 38.525 (Fig. 6.1).

© The Author(s), under exclusive license to Springer Nature Switzerland AG 2025   69
S. Satapathy et al., *Noise Pollution and Ergonomic Intervention by Acoustic Material*,
Synthesis Lectures on Mechanical Engineering,
https://doi.org/10.1007/978-3-031-66308-6_6

Table 6.1 Noise measurement before and after use of acoustics in a Drawing room

Room	Before condition	Noise in dB	After acoustics used dB	Noise in dB	Reduction in noise level dB	Outside noise 50 mm dB	After use of acoustic dB
12*12 square feet	Television running, trade mill	60	Wall	43	17	123	65
Door and window closed	Fan	47	Floor	40.5	6.5		
	Air conditioner working	60	Ceiling	40	20		
		55	Wall	50	5		

Table 6.2 Shape and size of acoustics basing on maximum noise absorbing capacity

Sound source	Noise In dB before placing acoustic material	Noise In dB after placing plane acoustic material	Noise In dB after placing rectangular acoustics	Noise In dB after placing cylindrical acoustic
Air conditioner	55	45	47	48
Fan	60	38	40	42
Grinder	87	80	82	83

Table 6.3 Perception of residential life after using noise absorbing materials

Sl no.	Question	0	1
1.	Noise level is reduced		
2.	No headache		
3.	Behavioral change occurs		
4.	No discomfort in hearing		
5.	Concentration level increases		
6.	No irritation		
7.	Work performance increases		

Table 6.4 Economic analysis of acoustic materials

Sl no.	Cost analysis		Qt	Unit price	Material requirement (1 sq. feet)	Price (rupee)	
1	Raw materials	Waste tire fibers	1 kg	30 rupee	50 gm	1.50	1.50
		Epoxy (L12) + Hardener (K6)	1.1 kg	708 rupee	50 gm	32	32
2	Overhead cost					(1.50 + 32)*15% (15% of material cost)	5.025
Total cost							38.525/-

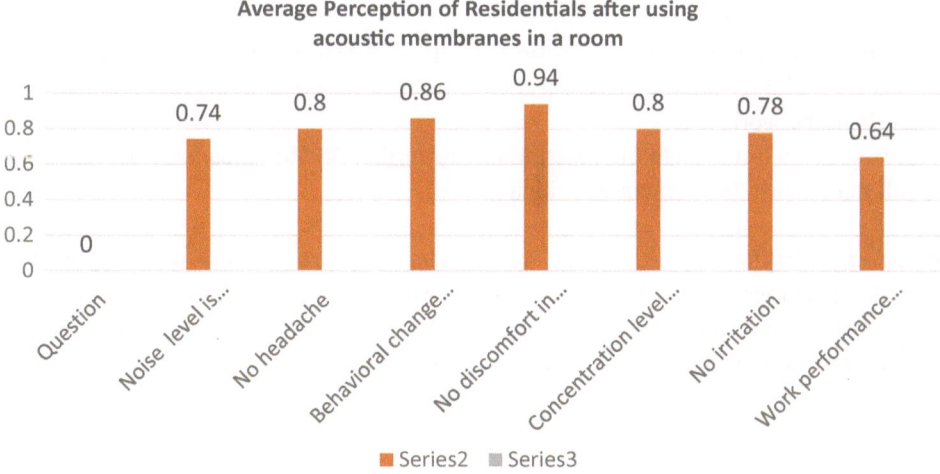

Fig. 6.1 Average perception of residential

6.2 Conclusion

Noise is the most persistent physical contaminant in the environment. Noise pollution is particularly prevalent in industrialized countries because of their social and economic structures, technological advancements, and population growth. In addition to noise pollution, occupational noise is also a major concern for workers. Noise pollution can cause hearing loss, disturbed sleep, cardiovascular disease, social disabilities, decreased productivity, unfavorable social behavior, irritability responses, absenteeism, and accidents.

Excess noise at the workstation was reduced using various processes. Among these processes, the use of an acoustic panel provides workers with a good and healthy working environment.

As is clear from the research, with the increasing population and rapid industrialization, sound has changed to noise pollution. By observing the negative effects on human health, the research suggests that their implications are necessary for society as well as the environment.

The implications of this research can be categorized for practical purposes, academics, researchers, and practitioners.

- This study will help other researchers to understand the importance of acoustic study and guide them to think and develop about new and alternate acoustic materials.
- This research will help researchers to understand about workplace discomforts and its negative impact on the body and mind.
- This study provides a platform for practitioners to design and modify workplaces to make them noiseless and comfortable for workers.
- It will also help to start new industries/startups to develop new types of acoustic materials for buildings and devices/instruments to measure noise levels and mitigate noise levels in the workplace.
- This study will also help the practitioners to further provide protective devices which will not disturb the workers with high noise

Moreover, policymakers, academics, researchers, and practitioners may frame rules/ suggest regulations against high noise and consider noise pollution as a serious issue. They must measure noise levels, suggest modifications, and take strict actions in every industry, academic institute, traffic place, and marketplace to avoid noise pollution rules.

Index

© The Editor(s) (if applicable) and The Author(s), under exclusive license
to Springer Nature Switzerland AG 2025
S. Satapathy et al., *Noise Pollution and Ergonomic Intervention by Acoustic Material*,
Synthesis Lectures on Mechanical Engineering,
https://doi.org/10.1007/978-3-031-66308-6